OUT OF THE NIGHT

OUT OF THE NIGHT

By
Clarence Crooms

VANTAGE PRESS
New York   Washington   Atlanta   Hollywood

OUT OF THE NIGHT

I have soaked in the hot springs of Arkansas, baked in the sun of Mexico and swum in the salty seas. I have been bound from head to feet with mustard plaster soaked in sea weed and peach tree leaves. I have swallowed every home remedy medicine I can think of and rubbed with every liniment—even the ones my dad bought for the plow mules.

I have buried myself in the earth hoping it would drown the pain out. Many times I have bitten my finger or lip to transfer the pain from one spot to another.

I have had a vision of heaven and a visit to hell. In the early years of my life, I would have been willing to be boiled in oil if I could have been free of the pain brought on by the illness that owned me.

I have prayed to die and still lived. I have prayed to live and died a little every day.

I have enjoyed some of the beauty of life and often bathed in the ugliness. I have always sought the tomorrow that would be better than the day I had today.

There is still no stop button for the treadmill I have ridden since the day I was born.

I do not know how long God will sustain me through

*the obstacle I have faced. I must write this account of my
life so that someone might obtain some degree of courage
and inspiration while encountering the same struggles.*

According to all medical reports and advice I have received, I have already lived a comparatively long life. *I
have sickle-cell anemia.*

I was born February 2, 1920 to sharecropping parents,
the eleventh of thirteen children, eleven boys and two girls.
I will name my family so that their names will be known
when mentioned in the story. My father: Alonzo, mother:
Indiana. My brothers and sisters in order of age are: Willie,
Lawrence, John, Bessie, Sarah, Richard, Lonnie, Amos
(who had sickle-cell anemia also), Bruce, Charlie, Clarence
(me), George, and James. We were all together only twice
ever, once when we had a family reunion and the other at
the funeral of my mother.

In those early years of my trials with my illness it was
called everything but what it really was, no one knew what
to do for it or about it. Some of the names given to it were;
spells, fits, even hoodoo. Mother was often told we were
"fixed." Naturally, I was born with this condition but
started to remember the dreaded attacks at age four.
Mother brought me up-to-date on the first years when I
was older. They were as dark and devastating as those I will
recount for you.

Medical attention for blacks was very poor in the
south, and to further complicate the problem we lived on a
farm four miles from the nearest doctor, who was white and
did not particularly care to come that far to attend a child
he thought might have eaten too much and had a king-size
stomach ache. He often told my parents to give me a dash
of epsom salts, baking soda, or whatever, and I would be
alright the next day. Being a wonderful mother as she was,
she tried them all at one time or another, but to no avail so
far as the pain in my body was concerned. I often screamed
all day and all night when an attack came upon me. No one

got any sleep during those times. Dad would go into the little town and get a small bottle of red medicine that was supposed to ease the pain. By the time the pains subsided everyone in the house was thoroughly worn out. This was a disadvantage I created for them because they worked in the fields from sun up to sun down to make the land give up enough to feed the family.

I knew of mother and dad's concern when the time came that I must go to school. The nearest school was an old church three or four miles away across fields, through marshy wooded pastures. There were no buses or other transportation for us in those years, so it was necessary for me to walk over the hills and through the marshes along with the others, sometimes lagging far behind even though they walked slowly and carried my books. They sometimes had to leave me behind because they would be late for school themselves.

When the dew was on the grass I would be wet to my knees because the path we took across the pasture was only as wide as we had made it by walking that way daily. I was seldom included in the games at school, my older brothers thought I might have a "spell." Playing the games might not have helped me any, but the attacks came whether I was sitting quietly in the school room or under a shade tree at home.

I was able to go to school a little more than half the usual time, but through reading at home and doing assignments sent to me by the teachers I was able to maintain a good average.

When school was over the young ones would join the farming chores, chopping cotton, pulling grass and the many other chores that go with farming I am afraid I did not live up to my father's expectations on the various chores. In south Georgia, when the weather was hot, it was very hot and when it was cold I had trouble even going to the henhouse in the backyard. Either temperature so often proved too much for me, I would have to retreat to the

shade, the fireside and sometimes to bed for days with
another attack, the same painful days and nights I had
known before. I could not sleep and did not feel like eating. My mother or one of my sisters often force fed me
with chicken broth or any kind of fresh fruit they could use
to keep me from starving.

With no medication available an attack might last ten
days. Those were days of pure agony and frustrations. The
other children were going about their work or play as usual,
I was all alone except for mother doing what she could to
make me comfortable. Even her best efforts proved to be
very little, she did not know what to do nor did she have
anything to do with. Her motherly love and fervent prayers
were my only solace. I often saw the tears before she
brushed them away with small hands well-worn with house
work and the toil of the cotton fields. I say here, without
reservations, she had to be the best mother in the world,
she gave birth fourteen times and raised thirteen children
to adulthood.

*I remember very well when I was thirteen years old en-
tering high school.*

I went to school that day feeling as well as I ever felt
in those days, it was a beautiful September day, the woods
were still green and wild flowers were still abundant. We
went on a kind of field trip through the woods, picking
flowers, looking for odd rocks, swinging on low tree branches
and whatever else we could do to have fun. We had walked
and played until we were a mile or more from the school
building when clouds began to gather and thunder began to
crash heavily. We had started walking back towards the
building when the rain came down so heavy we could
hardly see our way down the road. We started to run as fast
as we could to get back across the foot bridge because when
rain came down so fast it often pushed the little bridge
right down the stream with it. As we ran my heart began to

pound so rapidly, I felt as though it would close my throat. The extreme acceleration of my heart started my body aching from head to foot. I was so exhausted I fell flat on my face in the red clay mud and did not have enough strength to get up, much less continue across the flooded creek. After helping the other small boys and girls across, two of my brothers came back for me and put me on a board pew in the back of the church building. They knew they could never lug me home so one set out on foot to get mules and a wagon to take me home. While walking those three miles, then driving a team of worn out plow mules back, even a longer way than he had to walk, I was as ill as a little boy could be and still be alive. There are many descriptive adjectives in all languages but none in any language that can adequately describe the pain of a sickle-cell anemia crisis. No one, not even the doctors, could describe it unless he or she has it. Imagine having a toothache for four days without an available dentist and you will have a vague idea how a person with sickle-cell anemia feels in about an hour after an attack comes upon him. When my brothers returned to the school (church) mother was with them. She brought quilts, pillows, and a tarpaulin to cover me so that I did not get any colder or wetter than I already was. I had begun to scream, the pains were so severe I could not hold my peace. Even my teeth ached. Mother gave me hot chicken broth to help me to warm up; how she kept it hot I never knew. My brothers put me in the wagon wrapped in the quilts and blankets, my mother sitting flat on the floor of the wagon, with my head on her lap, constantly tucking the covers, wiping my tears and her own. The wind was blowing now, with a chilly fall breeze and even wrapped in all of the quilts and blankets I was about to freeze to death. Lying there in the bed of that old wagon, with the mules going about a mile per hour it seemed we were on the way forever. I felt every bump in the road and the pain penetrated my body like a rifle shot on every one. Mother's unwavering confidence that I would be all right was really something for me to hang onto; she assured me a thousand times that she was there and would never leave me; she said, "I am going to make you a hot tub bath, put you to bed and give you some more soup and hot biscuits."

My pains were so severe by this time it seemed to be pitch dark in the room even though there was a blazing hot log fire in the fireplace. I was trying very hard to soak myself in a number three washtub of hot water. I turned from side to side or into any position I could get into to soak the most of my aching body. Bessie brought me the soup and tried to force feed me, but one sip of the soup and my stomach rejected it along with everything that was sent down there within the last few days. Bessie asked, "Is that the way you are going to pay me for trying to keep you from starving?" She helped me into the chair in front of the open fire in order to change my bed. As I sat there completely engulfed with pain, I wondered which would be worse, to endure the endless pain or just a short plunge headfirst into the flames.

I pulled myself to a standing position in front of the fireplace. Immediately my homemade flannel night shirt began to smoke and the parts touching my flesh seem to blot out the pain temporarily. When I told my sister this, she got the idea to heat towels, clothes or anything she could use, wrap me into them then pull the covers up over them. The pain subsided and I slept until about four o'clock in the morning. I was awakened by an urging to use the pot—our toilet was an outhouse; therefore, we used a pot and delivered everything to the outhouse the next morning. I had perspired heavily while sleeping; therefore my shirt was wet and I became chilled while using the pot and the pains came back with a vengeance. Mother heard me rolling around in discomfort and came to me. She heated the towels and packed me back into bed, then she sat on the bed, rocking me gently and singing in a hushed tone, "I'll Overcome Some Day," "Jesus Keep Me Near the Cross," on and on. She asked me if I knew how to pray. I said I know the Lord's Prayer. "Yes, I taught you long ago," she said, with a deep look of sincerity on her face., "but I mean the kind of prayer when you really want something very special, something that means more than a bedtime prayer at night when you go to bed." I told her I had heard many people pray at church but did not remember what they said, nor what some of them meant. Mother said I should learn my own prayer, my needs were different from any I had heard.

I realized I must find a power greater than this evil demon within me. Medical care was so poor it was hardly worth building up hope seeking it. I began by asking the Lord for what I needed most; relief from pain and a degree of health so that I could play as the other children did, go to school regularly, and eat whatever we were fortunate enough to have. I often ate my dinner at four or five o'clock and lost it at six or seven, sometimes immediately. This crisis (I say crisis now, they called it spells then) lasted until the first week in October. I was very weak and worn when it was over; my strength had been completely drained. It came back slowly. My strong desire to return to school almost pushed me into another crisis before I was out of this one.

When I finally returned to school, some of the children whispered in small groups, making word bets that I would soon have another spell. I knew it would not be long, the crisis came very hard and very often in those years. I used to pray that God, through his mercy, would let me go through some special event. I would sometimes make it if I avoided extreme cold, heat or other aggravations.

Even though the depression was evident everywhere we always had fun on festive holidays. We had a turkey or roasting chicken from the barnyard, potatoes harvested from the fields, a Christmas tree from the woods. Those were days I sometimes relive in my mind, but I must continue with other accounts of my trials. I will not recall all of the crisis I have had over the years, for if I did I would have a book that would rival *Gone With the Wind* in volume. The circumstances surrounding them were good, bad and sometimes, pure *Hell*. I did not have a crisis during the holidays that year, everything else was about the same, the fruits (Nehi pop), the few gifts, were the same as the year before and would be the next year. There were about ten days until the bells rang again to start the New Year. I was looking forward to getting back to school and my friends.

The day we returned to school it was cold and cloudy, with winds that whipped the dry cornstalks making sounds like I had heard in ghost stories on the radio.

We started earlier than usual that morning so that I could get used to the distance again for the twelve hundredth time. I made it that day after what seemed an eternity. Time moved on; February, March, and April with the traditional showers. Farmers were planting new corps with visions of getting out of debt dancing in their heads, but I knew from the look on their faces that things worked out for most of them the same as last year, still owing two hundred and seventy-five dollars that might as well have been two hundred and seventy-five million—never quite enough. Dad was clearing new ground that year. The children had the chore of picking up branches, roots and other waste to be burned along the edge of the acreage. My brother, George and I started wrestling in the plowed ground and for the first and only time, I threw him flat on his back in the furrows. He started swinging a long flexible tree root that struck me in the back of the head. I wear the mark today. Dad gave both of us many lashes with a peach tree branch. All this overloaded my little wagon. By evening my lights began to go out. I was aching and my stomach was churning at forty miles per hour. I was hesitant in saying anything to anyone about how I was feeling. I kept praying it would go away and I could go to school the next day, but that was not to be. My arms and legs ached so badly I could hardly get ready for bed. I forgot the blow on the head, the steadily increasing pain elsewhere completely overshadowed it. The wound was treated only once with soap and water but healed all by itself while I went into another deep "spell" (crisis). Some of the children who went to school down the lane from our house said they could hear me half a mile away screaming and praying that God would ease the pain. Dad sent for the doctor after two days of this torment. The doctor came and gave me paragoric and left some to take later. I had always thought paragoric was for babies—now I knew. It did not touch the pain one little bit in the dosage he prescribed but I could only have it every four hours—every eternity as I saw it, minutes hung on like hours.

Soon the April showers had passed and May flowers were here.

My suffering continued, the pain seem to have taken up eternal residence in my bones. The school year was coming rapidly to a close. They closed on June first come fail or whatnot. This was a source of concern for me. I was concerned as to whether I had enough time in school to pass to the next grade. Slowly my latest darkness came back to light. I went back to school three weeks before it closed and was happy that I received a promotion. We had a closing program that included songs by the choir, recitations and a short play of the Uncle Tom type dialogue. When the program was over the students stood at attention while the few whites, who had the best seats, filed out to their automobiles and drove away with a familiar smile on their faces. The Uncle Tom play had shown them that the Jim Crow situation was still well in hand.

June came so beautiful, with blossoming trees, the pastures resplendent with green grass and wild flowers.

The streams running through the woods were so clear, one could often see small fish swimming up and down searching for food. You could see the polished stones at the bottom of the streams. I used to sit and look into those streams and make up imaginary cities in far away places I had read about, especially of Egypt. The large stones were the Pyramids, the smaller ones the homes and inns, and the flat sand beds the deserts. I often read books when I felt better after a crisis. Many of those far away cities were very real to me. They took me on trips around the world by boat or hiking, or swimming in a tropical stream.

The days of June were waning, farm chores were in full swing, something for everyone to do.

There was grass and cloves to be pulled from the cottonfield, and pigs to be fed. Sometimes the well ran low and water was brought down the hill from a spring. We also took the animals down to the spring to drink. Some of the mules often became frisky and would run into one of the fields. The tobacco field was the nearest and dearest to my father. It was called the money crop and just one broken stalk was a waste. It was one of those days in July that, while watering the animals, one high spirited mule ran through the tobacco field with all of us in hot pursuit I really mean hot. The temperature stayed between eight-five and one hundred degrees during July and August, especially at midday. The sun came straight down and there were hardly any places to hide from it. We finally caught the mule without too much damage to the tobacco. After the chase my brothers decided to go to the swimming hole. I hated being left out of everything so I persuaded them to let me go along. We were even more exhausted when we reached the swimming hole, it was more than a mile away. We did not have or need swimsuits. So, as we hastily peeled off our sweaty overalls and shirts we went plop, plop one after the other into the cool, clean creek water. I swam for a short while then sat on the sand of the creek bed where the shade of the tall pine trees was coming over me. I brushed away the sand from my body and pulled my faded overalls on. The others were still swimming and having fun, playing games in the water, but I knew the games were over for me. The sudden changes from hot to cool then back to hot from rolling in the sand had been too much for me. I had to walk the distance back to the farm house before I became too weak and pained. As I walked I sought strength from God through prayer. When I was alone I said many pleading prayers aloud. *God don't let it get me down this time. I want so much to be well, there are so many things I want to do, please help me fight.* Even though I did not know what I was fighting I believed God would help me, as I still believe today. In spite of my prayers and pleading my attacks took me to the very fires of hell. Only God brought me back with more determination to fight. For the present my fighting power was fading and by nine o'clock that night my lights were truly out; my suffering was beyond any description I can make here. My legs, arms and back were as stiff as iron bands. I could not pull the covers up if I was cold or down if I was hot. There was a small portion of the red medicine left from a previous time but it seemed to accelerate the pain.

Everyone did his share in trying to help but I was already in a bottomless pit fed by flaming fevers that tugged at every fiber of my body. My screaming was enough to keep the devil and his disciples awake for a week. The pain and the screaming exhausted me completely. I hardly knew what was happening around me. After about six days, my darkness began to lift, I could move my arms and legs and take some soup I asked my sister Bessie what day it was and she said, "Six days from the old swimming hole."

Mother and Bessie placed hot towels on my back to get it workable again. My spinal column seemed to get more damage out of this crisis than any other part of my body. For many weeks it was sore to the touch. There were many days, though, no one knew that but me. I was hesitant to try to sit or walk because of the stabbing pains in my back. The other children wondered why I did not go to the fields or play games with them at evening time, but I am sure my mother knew, she always knew. I was always glad to take cool water to the fields or anything I could do to be doing something helpful. I always feared becoming an invalid with nothing to do but vegetate and wait to be struck down even further than before. I know now that only by the mercy of God I came back again and again, kept living, and had some degree of happiness with my family and friends.

Doctors often told my parents they did not know what kept me alive. The only children they knew with symptoms similar to mine were long since dead. Of course, all the children were black and had very little medical care, the same as I.

I could see the concern on my parents' faces. Mother always said she was not going to lose any of us until we were grown but I am sure she sometimes had doubts about my brother Amos and I. He also had sickle-cell anemia, but did not suffer regular attacks as I did. He was able to live a much more normal life than I in those early years. Amos had leg ulcers and constant stomach aches but no one linked them to sickle-cell anemia. I tried hard to be normal; I was as daring as anyone. I would run a race, ride a horse at full speed, or swim across a creek. But the price I had to pay spiraled like a black cloud before a hail storm.

I grew up slender and tall with black wavy hair that most girls would like to have had. Many people said I looked girly, which burned me worse than the pains ever did. Mother's friends said that, "If he was a girl he would not have those spells." Cottonpicking time was upon us again, with white fields as far as the eyes could see. I looked across those fields and wondered how many days of back breaking toil were there. Although many of my brothers and my two sisters could gather two or three hundred pounds a day, dad brought people from town to help with the harvest. After many days of early mornings and late evenings the white fields turned to black empty stalks, except for a few late opening holes which were speckled in the black like snow flakes in a cool yard. Those few scattered scraps were an unpleasant chore of the younger children. We scrapped cotton here and there until late October, when we came home from school it was necessary to pick a burlap bag full of cotton before it became too dark to see. That bag full of scraps amounted to about two bushels, so you can imagine how far one has to walk to get that many scattered holes; ten or fifteen feet apart. There was one other chore we had in those days that boggles my mind to this day, that was gathering velvet beans. (I do not know their proper name velvet beans were just what they were called.) A pod about three inches long coated with a velvet-looking fuzz that fell off when they were touched after ripening. This velvet substance caused severe itching on any part of the body touched except the palm of the hand. They were planted in the cornfields and ran up the cornstalks often pulling the corn to the ground. It was next to impossible to gather those beans without striking our arms with the fuzz. If we were not extremely careful we sometimes leaned against other vines striking our neck against a bunch of beans. It would itch until washed off with soap and warm water and greased with Vaseline.

After chores like those I often had a restless night, many nights getting no sleep at all. The distance to school was already difficult enough for me, so after an exhausting evening and a sleepless night it was next to impossible. I remember one of those mornings mother was standing outside when we started on our way, my progress was so slow she called me back; she knew I would never never get there on time and would slow the progress of the others. I was disappointed, I enjoyed school and knew even in those days that I must get an education if I was to survive. I knew I could not earn a living doing what my brothers were doing farming, railroading, some collected the pine tar from the pine forest. I must learn something less physical.

Thanksgiving was about ten days away and the gathering of pumpkins and potatoes was a time we all enjoyed. We often had some still in the field since Georgia weather was not so severe. We had contests to see who would bring the pumpkin that would be used for pies. One of my older brothers generally brought back the right one, the good ones were larger than I could carry so I never won the contest.

Festive holidays were something to look forward to at our house my mother was a champion soul food cook, when the word soul was still thought of as the eternal spirit that returned to God when one died. There were no cans to open, no boxed pie crust or cake mixes and no gelatin substances for fancy salads. The cakes and pie crusts were made from the wheat of the fields, the stuffing from meal ground at the old mill on the pond. Pie filling could be any fruit your appetite might call for at the time. There were also some vegetables that could be made into pies. Many of those fruits grew on or around our farm land. Turkey, ham and chicken were in good supply. After a dinner like that we all should have had to go to confession, we had sinned most grievously.

For November, the days were beautiful, but there was winter chill in the air and enough wind to rustle the naked pecan trees in the back yard. I sat on the side of the table near the warm stove eating an extra piece of potato pie when I felt warm tears down my cheek. My world seemed to stop right there. I felt a crisis coming on. I wondered, why me—why now? I let more tears come; for the first time in my life I was feeling sorry for myself. The holiday was just beginning and I was already a dropout. They bundled me up and put me to bed, but I was already on that one-way elevator going down into a darkness blacker than a thousand midnights. I fought back with all I had and said all the prayers I knew but the battle was soon over and my strength was limited and God knew how much I could bear and stayed out of it.

The doctor was called but this was one of the times he

chose to come at his own discretion, which was four days later. He came in huffing and puffing as though he had walked the four miles from town instead of driving his dilapidated T-Model Ford. I was pushed down flat in the bed, then he went through his usual routine of taking my temperature, pulse, listening to my heart and thumping my stomach. He handed me a pill of some sort and was gone in less than ten minutes. I felt worse than I did before he came and pounded my stomach. My stomach boiled up so high till I was no longer able to retain its contents. I delivered it over my bed and the floor. My head whirled like a spinning wheel. I thought I would surely die here and now. Fortunately the doctor was still in the neighborhood and my father called him back when he had finished his other calls. This time he wiped my arm with a piece of cotton, still set from one of his other patients, and gave me an injection. He said to my mother he was sure this would keep me quiet for a while. I came out of it two days later feeling much better; most of the pain was gone. I felt so much better until I wanted fried chicken instead of the soup I always had.

My strength had gone down to the point that it was difficult to stand or try to walk. My strides were like a baby learning to walk for the first time. Mother encouraged me to keep trying every day, so I soon became stronger. By the time I was able to return to school it was almost Christmas. I think the distance between our home and school must have grown longer during that last illness. The cold winds beat about my frail body, chilling me to the bones. I wore as many clothes as I could successfully walk with, but walking through the open pastures and roads on my way to and from school, I might as well have been in the nude. I asked mother why she told my teacher not to let me play outside and she said I needed all my strength to get there and back. The other children played baseball most days; it seldom became too cold for them. There were many days of 70° weather even in December and January. I was envious of those strong healthy children, able to romp, race and play any game they wanted without fear of illness later. The inevitable consequences of strenuous play had now become frightening to me, so I turned my attention to books and games I could play without too much exertion.

At times this was very dull but I refused to become discouraged. In those days boredom was my constant companion. I was a charter member of Dullsville.

It was Christmas again. The berries on the holly trees were red, the pines were dropping their last cones on the grass that had turned brown and deposited their seeds for a more lush pasture next year. Walking through the woods I wished that things were as well with me as with the natural transfers that took place there. The changes there were automatic, from spring to autumn to fall without difficulty— "no pain, no strain." We had a good Christmas that year, not many gifts, as always, but we had a lovely holly tree in the middle of the room, plenty of food and friends, who came by to share food and friendship.

We had a fireball throwing on Christmas Eve night. Fireballs were made from scraps of clothing worn out during the summer harvest. The rags were rolled and sewn into balls then soaked in kerosene for several hours. When it was time to play the game the balls were squeezed out of the container and the excess fluid allowed to dry off. The balls were lighted with matches and thrown back and forth between players. If you could have seen that out where there were no lights you could never forget the beauty of it. It was hard for me to restrain myself from the activities, but I had come to realize the price to pay later for those few minutes of pleasure. As I watched the lighted balls fly back and forth in the darkness of the field I began to reflect back on the reason for the holiday we were celebrating. I remember the star that lighted the skies over the fields where shepherds watched their flocks on that night so long ago, when Christ was born. I could see the baby in the manger and the wise men who traveled far to pay him homage and bring gifts. I wish I could have preserved that night on film but had neither film nor camera. While watching all that and following my dreams, If I could have flown far away and never returned to the difficulties of my life I would have been very happy. Mother called to me from the doorway to come inside before I became chilled. I came in and closed the door on the fireball players and my peaceful dreams. It was back to reality for me. I did not sleep immediately because I could still hear the merriment outside the old farm house, the laughter and singing of carols as though they were in the next room. The fun lingered through the night.

My older brothers always brought fireworks to set off on Christmas morning but the younger ones were not allowed to play with them for fear of getting hurt. My father also protested vigorously against them. He said they should be set off on July Fourth to celebrate independence and not to disturb the peace on earth that Christmas represented.

I shall never forget that New Year's Eve. Clouds hung heavy and black as if it would snow. They seemed to burst into flames and the rains came down for nearly two hours as though it was attempting to wash away the toils of the outgoing year. When the thunder, rain, and the lightning were over a strange yellowish moon shown over the fresh countryside lighting the landscape almost as clearly as high noon. As we gathered in front of the big open fireplace and sung the old year out we could hear guns going off at the distant farm homes—their way of bidding good-by to the old year and greeting the new. If my story sounds like a vicious circle or repetitious that's because it is just that. Growing up for me was crisis after crisis and the events that preceded and followed.

Time moved on for me, sometimes swiftly, sometimes slowly, according to the state of my health. If it was good today it might be bad tomorrow and worse the day after that. The grim spectre of sickle-cell anemia has haunted me doggedly every day of my life. But for the strength God gave to me and the loving care of my family during my young years I believe my life would have been much shorter. It could not have been any more difficult; God's mercy and sheer determination are the key words to any reasonably active life with this monster on my back. Fear and agitation are devastating accessories to the crimes of Sickle Cell Anemia. I prayed every day for just one more chance to overcome. I felt the compassion of God's blessings some of those days and felt left out on others. My peace is as a morning cloud. Like the dew that goes early away. My parents decided I should live in town for the next school year. The distance I had to walk from my home continually plagued me. I missed many days I could have gone if the distance had been shorter.

As I grew older the crises seem to come upon me without provocation.

I often had them in class and had to be taken home by some of the boys in my class. I did not have as much of a problem getting a doctor since I was there with my sister and later with my brother Lonnie and his wife Arie. Lonnie worked away from home for the Seaboard Airline Railway Co., so Arie would get the doctor then send a message to the family that I was ill again and what she had done to make me as comfortable as was possible.

My mother would get one of my brothers, who by this time had their own automobile, to bring me home as soon as possible because she knew I would embarrass Arie by alarming the neighbors. Some of them were genuinely concerned and came to see if they could help Arie with anything. I could see the look of disbelief in their eyes because many of the housewives had seen me go off to school or down to the store perhaps two or three hours ago. The neighbor's small children would shy away from that home.

They said, "That boy is over there having another fit." I had began to learn how to control the outward screams but on the inside the fury was like a raging forest fire consuming everything in its path. I have cried many times, *Oh God please take me away, hide me until this is over, for I shall not be able to stand it much longer.* I often became delirious and said many things that my mother did not seem to understand. I also saw many things while not delirious that my family could not understand—I saw long roads lined with beautiful trees and flowers, lighted by hazy blue lights. I saw peaceful valleys with cattle grazing and horses running in the dust created by the wind. I believe that God was showing me there was peace in the world but for some reason I had very little of it. This did not disturb my faith in God. I know that without him I would surely lose my battle, and become more of a burden on my parents.

I believe that I had some thoughts, insight and communication with God I would not have had, had I not been ill. I was never fanatically religious, but knew that God was, and is, my saving grace. Due to being shut in so much, my dreams, subconscious, when I was asleep and my daydreams were very vivid. I chose to call them day-dream thoughts. They came into my mind like poetry, although not in verse, just beautiful words like this:

Death I do not fear thee. I would consider thee a sanctuary—I do not beckon thee, but if this is my lot I shall not shrink, I will not whimper, I accept the wish I no longer linger here. My heart is heavy and my body is drowning in pain. I see lands far away that are not troubled, mountains covered with snow swept by the winds. I see valleys green with grass—dotted with trees to shelter those who might come here for rest. I saw skies of blue, flowers, clouds of gray, rain, hail, rivers and streams—running like silver ribbons through the thick green forest. I heard music, the soft beating of many drums, the chimes of the organ in the clear morning air.

It came as though from Heaven, drifting through my open window. There were no lyrics, no theme, just beautiful music.

I did not know I was in a land of restrictions—the deep south. I did not know this was a land of oppression and deep depression. My heart sand songs of joy—the songs of Zion. I felt there was a Mecca for me somewhere and I bowed my head to the rising sun and was at peace with everyone. I must not let myself go so far from my illness because it is still very real. However far my thoughts may have taken me I must return to reality. I can not accept (until today) the theory of the most learned doctors that I would surely die by the age of thirty-five years or less, although I have been told this for almost thirty-five years.

Through many years of pain and struggle I have now reached my junior year in high school.

I thought that after moving to town to atttend school I would not be exposed to the cold weather, the long walks and the field chores, I would not have sickle-cell crisis as severely as before but I was very wrong. One of my most severe attacks came on at the school's field day and picnic. This was a very gala event for the school and from the very first plan for the function everyone looked forward to it with wild anticipation. I went to school early that morning dressed in my picnic clothes, ready for the fun and games. We did not have very far to go to the Old Roundtree Park so we walked along in class order, boys and girls separated.

We arrived at the picnic grounds about eleven o'clock and the fun began. I could not participate in the games but enjoyed the fun of them. We had potato-sack races, jump-rope contests, relay races and many others. The girls and their mothers had cooked foods to fit the appetite of any king. The principal called a recess in the games and everyone came to get food. Some boys and girls coupled off in different spots. I was sitting on the grass with Lillian, a girl I was very fond of. We ate and talked about school, movies and other things teenagers talk about. It was a beautiful day in May, not a cloud, no cares, no worries. I was happy and having the kind of fun I liked until suddenly it seemed to get dark. I felt as if the lights in my body and soul were slowly going out. Voices around me seemed to be yells. Some of the children were playing baseball and the crack of the bat against the ball sounded like thunder. I turned flat on my back on the grass but felt I was lying across stones pushing up through the ground. I did not scream out loud, I did not move. Lillian kept calling to me, asking if I was alright. Her voice was loud and clear but I could not answer, my diaphragm seemed to be choking me to death, my rib cage seemed to collapse around my heart and lungs, not allowing enough room for breathing. As I lay there the pain came on stronger and stronger. My strength ebbed away like water poured on hot sand. My breathing came hard because of the terrible pain in my ribs and chest bones. I was there on the ground for about half an hour but for me it seemed like 20 days. The fun and games were over for me almost before they had begun. I whispered aloud, "Oh God, why me, why now?" Lillian put her hand over my mouth when I cried aloud and said in a hushed voice, "It is not only you, it is me, too, and all of your other friends. We all wish we could help. We cry in frustration because we love you and are unable to help." I will never forget those words she said that day. Her concern and that of my other friends was a great consolation. They left me feeling as though I had allies to help me fight back. The boys took me to Lonnie and Arie's home and she called the doctor for me. Doc said he would give me a small shot of morphine but he thought it would not do much good. It didn't.

Lillian was a senior and would be graduating in June. I

feared I would still be flat on my back and would miss the graduation dances and parties that always followed. I began to recuperate slowly. My trips back from the volcano of hell had become longer, every day was forever, nights were never over. I could not sleep. My mind wandered into beauty that seemed fantasy but for me was an escape. Sometimes I wandered through fields of clover, sometimes in peaceful valleys. I often sailed to far away lands, hoping that somehow I could escape the agony of aching bones and sore muscles. I hoped that when my mind returned to my body it (my body) would be whole again; my longing for a normal life was stronger now. There were so many things I felt I was missing. I was afraid to go very far away where perhaps no one knew me, or would be afraid or unable to help me. My knees were still a little shaky but I attended the graduation. The girls were crying from joy, the boys were sad because they would probably never see some of those beautiful girls again. I do not magnify the severity of my sickle-cell attacks nor my fights to survival, I do emphasize the fact they were never-ending struggles. I sometimes lost as much as twelve pounds during an attack. In my wandering mind I had no fear of losing my battle to sickle cell, in reality I had my doubts as various times.

I attributed my ability to come back after an attack to my ever increasing faith in God. There was no medication to help me back because the doctors did not know what had happened to me in the first place. The pills and injections given me by them was an attempt to kill the pain, they were not very successful because they didn't know what caused it or how severe it was. The doctor said he could not find anything in his medical books that would cause that kind of pain in every bone of a person's body, he could only take my word for it. I remember a doctor having a medical clinic and workshop in Lyons, Georgia, and the doctor who had attended me many times discussed my case with the others. They set aside one day for "Coloreds" and asked my father to bring me down so that they could examine me.

He took me down early one morning so that he could get back to his farming, but it took all day. I was told to take off all my clothes and remained that way all day. I went through every test they could think of. I even walked a yellow line similar to what was used to determine sobriety after an arrest. I also ran the fifty-yard dash; there was plenty of space for it because the colored program was held in a tobacco warehouse. (The tobacco was still there.) After walking the line and running the 50-yard dash they would listen to my heart again and again. After each examination they would shake their heads as if I was something very strange. They took blood samples but after examining them several times failed to notice the odd-shaped cells. The doctors punched and probed, and drew blood until I felt I was an experimental cadaver. They asked me to drink a liquid that tasted like vinegar mixed with ale. I drank as much as I could but they were never able to complete that examination because the liquid came back so quickly until I had to catch it in the tin cup I drank it from. They seemed discouraged with me and told me to get dressed. I was so weak that my dad had to help me to get my clothing. They called my father into a small office to talk with him about the tests they had completed so far, and told him they would tell him about the others when they were finished.

In a few weeks we received a letter from Savannah concerning the other reports. My mother read the letter to my father and me. They stated frankly that there must be something wrong with me mentally, since they did not find one single thing that could cause the attacks I had. They recommended I be taken to Savannah to see a psychiatrist if we could afford it. If we couldn't pay, then I should be taken to Milledgeville, the state mental institution and let them take me through a series of tests there. When mother had finished the letter she ripped it into small shreds and burned it in the cooking stove. Then she said, "Lord I don't want him put up like that. They would let him die when he got sick again. Lord I will take care of him, just give me the strength I need, I'll take care of all my children till they can help themselves." When she became worried she would sing. "I'll overcome some day, I will not yield, I'll overcome some day." She would often hum with a heart-rending tone I have never heard from anyone else. The troubled look on her face during these times would shame the devil's alliance with sin. I do not believe the depth of trouble in her heart could be measured by man. Only God knew the turbulence within her and only he had a medicine to soothe it. I think Thomas A. Dorsey wrote the prescription for her heartache many years ago:

> Precious Lord, take my hand, lead me on, help
> me stand;
> I am tired, I am weak, I am worn.

I was no longer a child now but the prayers, the reverence, and Godly force with which she fought for my life and well being remains heartwarming and inspiring to me until this day. There was a strength in her never matched by anyone I have ever known; yet to see her she was delicate, fragile and very beautiful. I do not lavish praise on her because she was my mother, I only relate the true qualities she had that gave us all an inner push we would never have had had she not instilled it in us while we were young. She would say to us, if you are going to do a thing, you must put everything into it necessary to make the end results worthwhile. If anything defeated her she would say, "Lord knows I tried." I remember the day she received a letter from St. Louis stating Lawrence had some difficulty with the police, we were butchering hogs. She put the letter in her apron pocket and kept on working until late evening. After the work was finished, then she sat down and cried. I asked to see the letter the next morning and she said, "Don't let it bother you, I have turned the whole matter over to the Lord, and I am sure he will do whatever is necessary, everything is in his hands. I've told him what I want. Do you remember we read in the Bible that God

held back the sun till Joshua finished the battle of Jericho."
I have often tried to visualize what my early life would have
been like without her, I know now that most of my tasks
would have been insurmountable without the mercy of God
and the love of my mother. She was my salvation from total
collapse in those early years.

I have worked hard on conditioning my mind and body
to resist sickle-cell anemia. I have not been successful thus
far. I must continue, however, because it is beginning to
embarrass me more as I grow older. I was afraid to partake
some of the pleasures normal for a healthy young man. I
never doubted my ability but feared the aftereffects. I
thought of becoming a minister but abandoned the idea because I did not feel I could conform to the Protestant ideol-
ogy. There was too much emotionalism. I believed that
the proper approach to the presence of God was a quiet
one. My closest contact has been through silent prayer or a
song. My peace is like a morning cloud, Like the dew that
goes early away (Hosea 64).

In my peace and reverence I like to sing softly—
("Sweet Hour of Prayer")

> Sweet hour of prayer, sweet hour of prayer
> That draws me from a world of care and bid me
> at my Father's throne, make all my wants and wishes
> known;

I learned so much by attending church with my family.
I did not like the extreme emotional sermons for myself but
for my parents and the other older people it was, joy and
fulfillment, a chance to shed all the toils and sorrows of the
week, a chance to cleanse their minds of the cares thrust
upon them by the responsibility of large families with
meager means with which to take care of them. I have
often heard them say, "We won't have enough again this
year but God willing we'll keep body and soul together.
We'll make do with what we have."

Ordinarily my parents were not overly emotional but

during church services; I have heard them cry out at various times, "Yes, Lord, Oh yes Jesus, I hear you, I hear you, Lord, have mercy." I did not know what it meant at the time but found out later when my troubles multiplied or when the world seemed to be closing in on me. There have been so many days in my crisis-ridden life when I thought *this will surely be my last.* Then I cried out as they did, I moaned as they did, wrung my hands and walked the floor as they did (if, I was able to walk). This nurtured my faith in God, increased my strength to fight this chronic monster that has plagued me all my days on this earth and sought to destroy me.

This is my last year of high school and I have entered with all my thoughts on earning good grades so that I might have an opportunity to go to Georgia State College the next year.

The heavy hand of the depression still gripped the country (especially the South) so that it was difficult even for the best black student to go to college unless there was help other than from the family. Things went well for me the first of the school year. I had no crises that completely incapacitated me in those first four months. I had pains severe enough to give in but was fortunate enough to keep going. Thanksgiving and Christmas were beautiful as usual. Our tables were always bountiful. And my brothers and sisters who lived near enough to come were home for the holidays. Some brought their own little families, the grandchildren were always a great joy to my parents, they spoiled them as we never were. I have enjoyed the freedom of the last few months. My school work has been very pleasant and my grades are good. I knew my family had no money to send me to college but felt that in some way I would be able to make a way. I had talked to the principal about my particular situation to see if he could recommend anything. At that time Georgia State was an industrial college, including farming, and a dairy, so Mr. Dickerson told me if I was able to work on the farm or in the industry he would talk to the administration officers and see what could be done. This gave me something to look forward to and an incentive to keep up the good grades. In February we always had two holidays—Abraham Lincoln's and George Washington's birthdays. Lincoln's birthday came on Thursday that year so we had a four-day leave from classes. All students boarding or living in with relatives quickly took off for their homes in the surrounding areas. I set out on foot to my home on the farm. The weather was comparatively warm but cloudy and overcast. I was fortunate to catch some of the other students going my way so that I did not have to walk alone. We had fun playing a dribble game—to see who could dribble the longest distance without losing the ball. When my turn came I kept the ball for about a half mile, enough to start perspiring and became somewhat exhausted. I gave up the ball to a friend and we sat down beside the road to rest before we continued to walk toward home. After about ten or fifteen minutes sitting and talking, I began to feel stiffness in my back and knees. I stood and began to move slowly down the embankment where we had been sitting and knew immediately that I was in serious trouble because we were only about half way home. My friend knew it, too; therefore, he walked slowly with me. My steps were faltering, my progress towards home became more difficult with every step I took. After nearly a mile my friend suggested I sit down beside the road and he would go on and get someone to come back for me. I insisted I could finish the journey if he would bear with me. I wanted to prove to him and to myself I could do it. I summoned every ounce of strength I had left and walked on more slowly and laborously than ever. My knees had swollen as if to burst with the very next step I made. We were finally in sight of home, but with the pain completely engulfing my body, the house seemed so far away I could hardly see it.

My heart raced as though I had run the mile in four minutes; my breathing was difficult also. I think every bone I had had become involved by the time I finally reached the front porch. I was as glad to be there as a weary traveler having walked ten times the distance.

My mother took one look at me and began to prepare hot water and the nearest bed. In the meantime, she would look at me, as I sat there bent double with pain and ask, "Why did you do this to yourself and me? I would have sent someone to get you tonight. You might have lost a few hours here at home but I am sure that would not have been as bad as this." I did not answer. I did not know the answer other than I thought that since I had done so well recently, I could make it without so much difficulty. This crisis really came down hard on me. Nothing seemed to help. I returned to the deepest fury of a burning hell. The doctor had been there but the morphine injections he gave me were nothing more than a needle prick. The pain hung on unchecked for longer than I care to remember.

It is late March now; I've begun to mend slowly.

Although the crisis seemed to have been endless, the time had flown swiftly by. The pastures were green, some wild flowers were peeking through, and outside my window in our small peach orchard a few of the beautiful blossoms were beginning to burst into powdery pink. I looked out the window every morning before breakfast and did whatever exercise I dared do to get my strength back. The blossom unfolded daily until the peach trees all wore big umbrellas of pink blossoms. Had I been able to count them I'm sure there were a million or more. The fruit grew so thick until sometimes the trees broke down under the great pressure.

As soon as I was able to begin thinking objectively, my concern turned to my schoolwork, which due to my long absence from classes, had been neglected. I began reading and studying all the work I knew the other students had covered during my absence. Some of my friends brought my books and some of the various examination questions they had copied for me. There were only a little over two months to go before graduation. My concern was catching up enough to graduate with my class and go to college. My principal had obtained permission for me to go to Georgia State on a working agreement as soon as graduation was over. After this crisis had brought me down so far I had some apprehension about going away from home but felt I must. It was now or never so I asked and received permission to take exams on the previous two months' work.

It was difficult for me to keep up and catch up at the same time. It was necessary for me to take all the exams in one day in the library since the classrooms were occupied by the other students with their regular work. The librarian told me she knew this would be a difficult day for me but I should work carefully, read and reread my answers before turning in my papers, because that was the only time I would have. She evidently graded the papers as I finished them. When I was ready to leave for home she said not to worry about the exams as she was sure I had done well in all of them. I was grateful for that, so that my anxiety would not overcome me before I received my grades. I received my graded papers a few days later and they put me back on an even level with my class and in position to graduate along with them.

It is May now; plans for graduation are at a feverish pitch. Measurements for rings, caps and gowns, placements for participation in the various programs hold everyone's attention.

The pace was very hectic those last few weeks of school. I had to stay on the sidelines as much as possible, trying to be sure and be there for the important ending. We had a beautiful Sunday afternoon for the commencement address at the historic First Baptist Church. There was an air of accomplishment among the students, pride and tears of joy among the parents. Our purple and gold caps and gowns gave a striking contrast to the white-painted choir stand of the old church. Our class sang the tune "Smiling Through," which was composed by the class. To me it was sad enough for tears.

The entire program was very well arranged and executed. Our commencement speaker was a professor from Forsyth, Georgia, very eloquent and well informed. His subject, in essence, was when you start out know where you are going. He told the age-old story about the three men driving through town in their big automobiles throwing dust and dirt all over the place. The first man drove through town in a big rush and parked in front of the bank. The newspaper reporter asked him where he was going in so much of a rush. "I own this bank," he said, "and I was late for an important engagement with a client." The second man came down the street in a like manner and in a few minutes parked in front of the insurance company. The reporter asked him the same question he asked the banker. "This is my insurance company," he said, "and I have a very important staff meeting." Just as the others had done the third man came down and parked along the main street. The reporter repeated the question, "Where are you going in such a hurry?" He stated that he did not know why he was rushing or where he was going, he was just going with nothing specific in mind. Almost everyone laughed. A few reflected on the significance of the moral of the story. I remembered that story because there was somewhere I wanted to go, so much I had to do when I got there, my main concern was getting there. The professor went on to deliver a long message which included many pertinent facts about the life that we faced and the times in which we faced them. He said there were those sitting there who were not college material, there were those who could make it at Harvard but could not afford it, some would go back to the cottonfields from whence they came, and some, the more fortunate, would achieve success at their endeavors. He was right on every score. Some became teachers, preachers, social service workers, and nurses. Others migrated north into auto factories and steel mills, and there were those who were not able to fight their way out of deep stagnation. They were consumed by frustration and alcohol, which they drank much too often, trying to forget their plight. That graduation was a memorable one for me. I was the first of my immediate family to graduate from high school. The others didn't graduate for various reasons. All were capable.

After the program was over my brother, Bruce, took mother and I home. I sat in the back seat and as we rode along I closed my eyes and wondered out loud. *What it would be like to really go to college?* My mother said she didn't know but professor Dickerson had said I could go as a working student if she thought I could make it that far away from home. I knew she had given it a great deal of thought. She turned around in her seat enough to face me, looked at me and said she could not make the decision as to whether I should or should not go. She would help me however she could whatever the decision would be.

Apprehensions nagged me for a while but the inner drive to prove to myself and others I could do it outweighed the apprehensions. I suppose you could say my ambitions outweighed my common sense. After the suffering I had had some would have been content to fold up their tents and avoid anything that might cause more. I knew I must press on or else sickle-cell anemia would consume me. I would be cast into the already overcrowded sea of the disillusioned. There were already so many young blacks who had thrown in the towel before the first round was over. Most people in our town and surrounding communities knew me and about my illness. Some were pulling for me to do well; some thought I would not be safe away from home and expressed this to my parents. There were those who were envious because they had sons and or daughters who were in good health but were not trying to do anything.

I could not sleep that night; my thoughts wandered back over the years of my childhood. I remembered the silly games we played, the times we had, some good and some not so good. As you can see by my age I was a child of the depression. I was nine when the stock market crashed. I did not know at the time what it all meant. I only knew we didn't have as many cattle and hogs as before and wore our clothes and shoes longer. I learned later how difficult those times were for my people. They were already poor and this made them poorer, I believe the word was *destitute.* I saw grown men wearing rags and long faces. I remembered the story about the sad-faced boy who played the harmonica, his music was sweet, it cheered everyone around him, but his discontent was so deeply rooted within him he never smiled. So it was with those farmers. Some did not know where they would get the next meal for their families. Poverty was known by my family also, but in spite of this my father often shared what we had with others less fortunate.

Soon the sun was rising, I could see the soft rays through the windows, also through some wide cracks in that old farm house. The pleasant smell of bacon and biscuits cooking was already inviting me out of bed. I was up and dressed quickly. I did not realize before that I had not eaten since early Sunday afternoon. The graduation excitement had taken away my appetite. The fields were beautiful in June, the tobacco, corn and the endless cotton acres were all green. Everything looked very promising for a good harvest. There was not an awful lot of work on the farm this time of the year; the cotton bolls had not opened enough to start the laborous task of gathering it. It was near the end of the growing season but not yet harvest time. During my hours of reminiscence I had decided I must take the chance of going away to school. I talked to my mother about it and we began preparations for me to leave immediately so that I could do whatever I could as a working student to be ready for the September classes.

There weren't many clothes to pack, one pin-striped, dark suit; two "matchme" suits, one gray, one brown; two white shirts; plenty of socks, given to me at graduation; underwear; and hankerchiefs my mother had made. There was very little money—seventeen dollars and train fare to Savannah. It was necessary for me to take the streetcar to the campus. I had never been on a trolley before and was fascinated by it. I had often seen them in the newsreels at the movies. The little wheel on the cable did not jump off as I had thought it might.

It was late afternoon when I arrived on campus. The whole place seemed deserted. I walked around for a short time without the slightest idea of where I should go. Shortly a couple came by going in the opposite direction. They stopped to ask if they could help. Finding I was just arriving for the first time they directed me to the administration office.

I was registered, assigned quarters and duties. The registrar said that Professor Dickerson had called about me in complete detail so I was given duties in the dairy and very little out in the fields. I was grateful for that because I had just left the farm to seek knowledge. I felt it would take me away from farming forever. To come face to face with another farm at this time would have been just too much and no doubt a trauma that would last for as long as I lived. When I speak of these farming chores I should remind you this was an agricultural college, but agronomy was not the only subject. I was there to pursue the others. I already knew all I ever wanted to know about farming.

There was one bitter pill to swallow in being a dairy

worker—getting out of bed at five A.M. Time made that pill a little more palatable; the work there being the only means to an end helped also.

As time went by I became more adjusted to things around me.

I made friends and enjoyed the evening gatherings. Since it was the summer session, there were not many students there.

In those years college students did not have beer busts or pot sessions. They generally gathered at the coop house to have ice cream, punch or a sandwich and to talk with friends. I did not know how poor and underprivileged I was until I had attended a few of those gatherings. The clothes they wore, the places some of them had gone and the things they enjoyed, I had never heard of before. I was more anxious to join them than before; they were giving me an education without knowing. I could not join them for dinner, only ice cream or punch. I could not afford dinner. Many of them received money from home periodically. I knew I must eat my meals at the dining hall in order to hold my original seventeen dollars as long as I could for any emergency that might arise from my health problem. I had been nickle and diming for ice cream and punch already.

I wrote a letter to my mother to let her know that I was doing well so far. She must have been thinking of me. I received a letter from her as I dropped hers in the campus P.O. She did not begin by asking how I was or how she was doing. She began:

Dear Son:

I am writing to tell you to take care of yourself and pray that God will guide you through all obstacles. I pray every night you will stay well, I pray you will be able to hold out against the sickness that bothers you so often. It seems you have been gone so very long. You children keep me on my knees praying for all of you. You all are gone from me now, I am a little sad sometimes, but I thank God you are trying to do what's right. Please write me a letter soon. Pa and the others here send their love.

Write soon
Mama

If I had saved every letter she sent me I would have had a stack in a short while. I knew she must be anxious to know if I was well, so I wrote to her as often as I could.

Working in the dairy included cutting corn from the field for the cattle. It was in on one of those days I began to ache around the shoulders and down my spine. With much difficulty I made out the day. I was beyond exhaustion, if that is possible. I did not go to the dining hall to get dinner. I went directly to my room, got undressed and went down the hall to the showers. I stood in the shower with the water spraying over my aching body, as hard and as hot as I could endure. I stayed as long as I could stand the pelting and to my surprise I felt somewhat better. I went to bed and said every prayer I knew, finally going into a light sleep.

About two hours later I awoke and the pain was back in my abdominal area with vengeance, it was so severe, I started vomiting and thought I would never stop. George, a friend, gave me some baking soda in warm water that helped temporarily. I was grateful for even five minutes of relief that was about as long as it lasted. I could feel myself going into that deep torrid pit I had known so many times before, a whirlpool of blackness I could not avoid. I could hear my mother's voice calling encouraging words; even though she was nearly a hundred miles away I had counted on her over the years for care and prayer. The school physician came in the following morning and gave me a flea flocker shot that seemed only to anger the demon that was devouring me. Without mother there, my fight was harder than ever before.

There was no strength left in my body with which to fight back, I knew I must rely on my mental will to survive. I closed my eyes and said to the pain that engulfed me, "I will not give in to you, I will not surrender, I am going to hang on until I defeat you." I repeated those vows so long I began believing them. I began feeling better but my fight was far from over. My body was numb in some areas. My head throbbed as though I had been beaten. My legs seemed to have died, I could not will them to move. After several days my mental power was working. I could walk to the shower and stand long enough to spray myself with hot water. I did that three times daily. It was exhausting the first days but I began to feel much better and accomplished my shower without difficulty. *Thank God, thank God, my mind is defeating the physical pain, not blotting it out completely but the effort is worthwhile.*

I was much improved but when I had a crisis I never slept well. That night the songs, the music and voices I had heard many times before came back to me. As I lay there listening and my thoughts wandering, a voice called to me: "Come, I will take you to a beautiful land far away, you have never seen the beauty of this land, you have never heard the songs the voices there sing." The journey was through an endless mountain pass lined with clouds radiant with many colors. It seemed never ending. Someone was holding my hand. I grew stronger as we went along. I felt no pain, no sadness, only peace and joy. Temporarily I had escaped the physical chains that bound me to my troubled body. I had never felt this joy before. My heart was as light as the clouds about me. I heard music but there were no instruments; it was made by a million blended voices. The chimes rang within my very soul. In a green valley wider than I could ever tell you, I saw a host of people clad in robes of every color of the clouds I had seen before. There were no tasks to be done there. They sang the glory of God all day. There was no darkness there, only peace, only love and happiness. My heart sang the song of Zion with them. My eyes wandered to a far away hill that was brighter than any sunrise I have ever seen. The faces of the singing multitude were all turned to that hill. No one spoke a word, they only stood in reverence, clasping their arms across their chests and bowing towards the light on the hill. Then suddenly as the final curtain fell, it was all gone.

I have tried so many times to hear that voice again and heed it so that I could be taken to that land again but have never seen it again. I am not going to try to lead you to believe I have been to heaven in the wanderings of my mind. I can only relate to you the joy of a journey of a wide awake wandering mind.

Shortly after my wandering was over, my friend came into the room with a letter from mother stating she had dreamed I was ill but hoped her dream was not going to come true. I'm sure she would not be too surprised how true it was already. Her letter began:

Dear Son:

I dreamed you were ill and I was unable to help you. I am constantly praying for you, that you can stay well.

I am sending you this letter you received from the government, I did not open it because it looked like those Bruce and Charly received stating they had to go to the Army. However I know you will be spared that because of your illness.

I read in the *Atlanta Journal* that the war clouds, so long gathered over Europe are now spilling over into our country and they are having some trouble also with the Japanese. There are five of you in the age limit but I feel I only have to worry about four. I am sure whatever happens, God will take care of you all.

Please write soon, I have not heard from you in weeks.
Love
Mother

I opened the enclosed letter and read the "greetings" from Uncle Sam. I applied for a collegiate deferment and received one. In the meanwhile, reading the *Savannah Tribune,* I could easily see that the tempo of the European War was picking up. Several of the Slavic countries and France were in deep trouble, and military activities in this country had been accelerated. There were discussions going on between the United States and Japan, with no one willing to concede. I don't really know what the issues were, I only know the talks became somewhat stalemated.

There were young people there at school with high hopes, counting on what they could accomplish when they had completed their studies. I often prayed this would not be destroyed. There was laughter there, hard study and some tears. There was so much to be lost if we were involved in a world conflict. Yet, in contrast to the present, I knew there would be no objectors. I wondered why but the answer was obvious. We were all here seeking dignity and identity, if any man or power sought to destroy this then fight we must. Anxieites grew among the young men there as time went on with disturbing news from the war torn countries of Europe. I was not concerned too much for myself, I thought only of other young men everywhere. I was very doubtful I would ever pass any physical examination because by this time I had one of the predominate symptoms of full-sickle cell anemia, a calcified hip joint (on my right side). I did not have much of a limp then, one would not known unless I was watched carefully.

I did not go home for the Thanksgiving holiday so it came and went without much of the celebration and feasting I was accustomed to. I went along with some friends to a movie, then had some seafood at Tiby Beach. Seafood was so reasonably priced one could easily eat all he wanted for only fifty cents. I really ate more than I needed. In a few days classes and the general routine for everyone was back to normal. The weather there on the banks of the Savannah River was beautiful even in December. There was fog early in the mornings but it generally moved out to sea before midday to be destroyed by the breeze. December seventh was a typical southern winter morning, bright skies with a slight cold breeze blowing in from the vastness of a restless sea. No one seemed in any rush to get anywhere. Suddenly an announcer broke in on the musical program on the radio. "We interrupt this program to bring you news of bulletin importance, the Japanese government's airplanes have just attacked the United States naval base at Pearl Harbor." He repeated the bulletin several times.

I do not know how many bombs fell on Pearl Harbor, nor how many young men whose hopes went down with them, but there were many on both counts. Many of my friends started packing their things to go home. They knew whatever reason they had not been called could not exist any more in the face of the tragic thing that had just occurred. Most of us received notice shortly thereafter to report to our local board in our various hometowns. There were many tearful good-byes, many pledges to return as soon as possible and some impromptu weddings. I was not in the wedding group but was a full-fledged member of the tearful farewells and the pledges to return.

I reported to my local board in Lyons, Georgia, about five months later, still unruffled, believing without a doubt, I would fail the physical and return to school. To my surprise the examination they gave was so negligible, there were no failures. We were told to report back there in three days with enough clothes for three days. We were to be sent to Fort Benning, at Columbus, Georgia, for further physical examinations and possible induction. I went along undisturbed, believing I would surely fail a more thorough physical examination. The buses arrived at Ft. Benning about 9:30 P.M. that evening and we were led to a barracks building that looked as though it had been abandoned since the Civil War and they had hurriedly thrown some very skimpy bunks up so that we could bunk up there until morning. Dinner mess was long over and there did not seem to be any preparations made for us to have anything to eat. Everyone was starved and there were many requests for food. We were told we should have eaten before we left home, they were not expecting any recruits until early morning. We were not allowed to leave that dilapidated barracks building, but were fortunate enough to get some of the few regular soldiers who had been there a while to get some sandwiches for us from a restaurant not far from the post gates. That was just enough food to frustrate everyone but we managed to survive through the night. I do not think there was much sleeping anyway. Soon we heard a trumpeter blowing in the distant area. I had never heard taps before nor thought about it in one way or another. To me it was a very sad tone, that had no special significance. An old man wearing sergeant stripes and every other hash mark one could possible get, came in and ordered everyone into their bunks and the lights out. Someone called out from the other end of the building in a loud voice to ask who he was. He called out in a loud blast, including more profanity than answer, and said he was the caller's mother and father and if he did not shut up he would be treating him as though he—the caller—was his girlfriend in a hotel room for a specific purpose. Everyone broke into laughter but found very promptly that was the wrong thing to have done. The sergeant came back, turned on the lights and went into a verbal blasting liken unto preaching a shouting sermon at a camp meeting only he was the sole participant and the songs and prayers had been changed to gravel voiced shouting and profanity. As quickly as he returned and finished his barking he flipped the light switch off and was gone again. Everyone lay in shocked silence. I began to hope with all my being I would fail that physical. If this was any indication as to what the army would be like I was sure I wanted no part of it. The strange thing about this was that we were not even in the army yet. We said we would all say a fervent prayer that we would not be subjected to that person if we became soldiers. I think we all put his attitude on trial and found him guilty of being ignorant and too stupid to know it. Well enough to keep quiet so that others would not know. His (AQ) aggravation quotient was much higher than his IQ.

There was the trumpet man again, and he was coming in loud and clear, his tune more cheerful than before. However I still asked myself was this a summons to Heaven or Hell?

Thinking and wondering as I did I failed to see any heavenly aspects in the whole situation. In came the profane old sergeant again, his garrison cap so far to one side of his neatly groomed graying head you could see the shaven part on the other. He was so militarily orientated, he called out "Ten Hut." No one seemed to pay much attention. We had never heard the word before but he had heard it so much he thought the whole world knew what he meant. He was livid with rage when no one stood to attention or even turned to greet him. He called us all kinds of names—like dumb rookies and many others I can not relate here. When the raving was over he told us to line up by two's and led us to the mess hall for breakfast. We only had about twenty minutes in which to eat. I had finished before that time expired. I could only eat the bacon and drink the small glass of orange juice, just looking at the eggs and fruit made my stomach flip a little. The eggs were powdered anyway.

From the mess hall Old Sarge took us to the medical depot to go through the physical exams. We were herded into a small roped off area and when our names were called we had to step in lines by two. These lines moved slowly

into the building. As we entered the double doors we were
told to remove all clothing, and if we had any valuables to
hold them in our hands. There were some pathetic sizes in
that room of nudity. The athletic looking ones made you
want to laugh, the scholarly and flabby ones made you want
to cry. Everyone had gone through the lines of doctors
without incident until the end of the line. There I think any
red-blooded American young man, who came through the
examinations, must have gotten the shock of his life—the
last doctor was a white woman. Her specialty was to
examine the anus. I'm sure you remember that the armed
services were still segregated in 1942. This was an all-black
medical station, so what in the hell was a white woman
doing there looking and feeling up black behinds. There
were many red faces there that day. The laughing and kid-
ding afterwards kept my mind away from the gravity of the
war we had been assembled here to fight. I had not let myself believe I would pass the physical, therefore was never
up tight. During the course of examinations when asked
about the previous state of my health, I stressed I had an
illness that came upon me periodically and how devastating
it was. They thought I was just another joker looking for a
way out. The lab tested my blood but I was sure they were
checking only for syphilis and gonorrhea germs. They
thought all blacks had one or the other of those anyway—
five percent had it now and had it earlier in their young lives.
Some were sent back home, some were sent to the hospital
unit for shots and brought back to the examining area. After
three days of hustling and fussing around in the nude, the
day for separating the strong from the weak came, the day
of decision was here. There is no way to tell you the apprehension I felt that morning. The sureness I had felt in
the days passed that I would fail the physical began to turn
into doubt. I was sure now that in spite of the clarity with
which I had related my illness to the doctors, they did not
really hear me or cared less if they did.
    After reveille and breakfast the next thing we heard

was a blasting loud speaker directing all recruits to assemble in what looked like a red clay racetrack near the medical station. When the men came to give orders that day they must have left Old Sarge at home. These were young commissioned officers. They brought a long tug rope and stretched it down near the center in the space in which we were assembled. They carried clipboards with papers and records. One of the officers explained the procedure we were to follow that day—when they began calling names they would say to the right or left side of the rope. For a short time the names were running about even on each side. As they went along the traffic moving to the left side of the rope came almost to a halt, while the right side was overflowing. They were not calling the names alphabetically because I had not been called for either side. I got the idea the left side was rejects, although there were many very strong looking men over there. After noticing the healthy looking men on what I had figured to be the rejects, that lifted my hopes of going back home. I just knew if they found something wrong with them, they must surely have found my cracked blood cells and calcified hip bones. However, this was not to be, and as the calling of the names continued I was sent to the right side of the rope. The assignments were soon concluded and everyone stood mute waiting for the officers to render judgment. They walked briskly out to the center of the clay-topped field where a loud speaker had been set up to make the announcement.

One of the officers took the microphone and began by getting the attention of the men assembled. He did not say what we wanted to hear immediately, he talked about the war, why it was happening and what we were going to help do about it. Finally, he turned to the men on the left side of the rope and reprimanded them for being such poor physical specimens. He said they should return home and try to improve themselves; they might be needed later. He then dismissed them and turned to our side of the rope.

"You men are now members of the finest fighting force

in the world," he said. "You will be quartered here for about five days. You may spend three of those days with your families if you can get there and back within that time. You will then be sent to another fort somewhere in the United States for training. There is no point in asking where you will be sent, no one knows that until you arrive."

My heart had been sinking since I was directed to the crowded right side of that rope. Now it was all the way down to my pelvic area. My presence here plus having been actually inducted into the army was beyond belief. When we were dismissed I stumbled back to my barracks building in deep shock. My friends were preparing to get away as soon as possible to visit their families but until I was asked was I going I had not given it much thought. They kept telling me, get ready, get ready, we can make that six o'clock bus to Vidalia.

I remembered the good-by I had said to my family and friends, the hope in my mother's eyes that I would be back in a few days. She was sure I would not pass the physical. My girlfriends refused to say any serious good-byes; they also felt I would return after the examinations were over. I sat there still in a daze from the day's events and a thought came to me to let the parting from family and friends remain as it was. There were no tears, no sadness. I had rather remember smiles than tears, joy rather than sorrow. I told those friends waiting for me of my decision not to go home. They were surprised, but some said they understood. There were very few of the men who did not go; most of them for the same reason; they did not like tearful partings. When the humdrum and din of confusion was over we had dinner and I saw down under the nearest light to write a letter to my mother.

Dear Mother,

To my surprise I was accepted into the army. I am

sure everyone there will be as stunned as I am but I do not want you to be sad, I do not want anyone to worry about me. I know this will no doubt take me farther away from home than I have ever gone before. I will miss you most of all. I shall always go with God at my side. I will be with him and he with me even to the ends of the earth—not even the furious battle can stop that. I know that God will guide me and I will follow. There must be a grail for my quest of peace of body and soul. I know that the pains that have rocked my body will follow me wherever I go, but I shall not give in to it. I will fight as never before. I want to live on an equal basis with my brothers, and my friends back at school and these here who are so vigorous and able. The only way I can do this is to try and try very hard beginning right now. If I fail this test I feel I will be completely emasculated before my family and friends. God forbid this. Love to everyone. Please keep well. I will write to you as soon as I am stationed. I will be gone from here before I could get a letter from you.

Love,
Clarence

The five days' stay was almost over. Most of the newly inducted men had returned. Speculation on where we would be stationed began before we were ever assembled for instructions and orders. Personally I could not have cared less where we would go. We could not go any farther south; we were already in the middle of the worst state in the union so far as being segregated and deprived were concerned. I played a little comparison game with myself. I tried to figure whether I would rather be back home picking cotton under the blazing sun or here with a gun on my shoulder preparing to fight someone I had never seen or even thought seriously about before Pearl Harbor (never heard of Pearl Harbor before either). I didn't come to a clear-cut descision. The cottonfields had already robbed me of much of my dignity, and I did not know where the gun on my shoulder was likely to lead me.

The man with the horn, blowing the sad song, came on as usual that evening. The sound had barely died before the perennial screamer, the Old Sarge, burst in and turned on the lights yelling, "OK everybody up and dressed in five minutes and report to the drill area where you were inducted into the army." We were up immediately throwing on clothing, scrambling for shoes and hats. Most made it on time, but those who did not were throughly chewed out by Old Sarge. I think he must have anticipated some late arrivals because he waited at the entrance and let out a profane blast when they approached the drill field. After everyone had been properly accounted for we were lined up in drill formation and called to attention by a young lieutenant. He apologized for calling us out in the middle of the night, but said he found it necessary, since most troop movements were made during the night, when possible. We were assigned to a troop train with Pullman-like beds. In a short time an officer came in and asked for volunteers for KP duty. He pointed to me and seven others and said, you just volunteered for KP for every day you are on this convoy. I thought that was the nail that would seal my casket, the long hours on my feet doing work like I had never been subjected to before.

The train begin moving about two-thirty that morning. Those of us on KP asked could we lie down for a while before beginning our duties. We found we had no time to rest. We had never been assigned a bed in which to rest. Since this train had just returned from a trip it was necessary for KP duty to begin immediately. We were taken directly to the kitchen unit. There we met twelve more disgruntled rookie soldiers from the other end of the train. We were handed a list of things to be done in order to have breakfast ready for six hundred men by six that morning. I never saw that many eggs, prunes, grits and slabs of bacon in all my life. I was astonished at the ease with which the chefs prepared the food after KP crew had carted it from the storage area and placed it into position as instructed.

Our most difficult chore came when the men started coming in for breakfast. The food was served by the KP crew, each on a particular pot or tray. Some men were spoiled and choicy. They would want eggs, bacon, bread and prunes, but no prune liquid to touch their toast or eggs. Some wanted grits with extra butter and bacon. Having been told how to serve the food and knowing we must do it exactly that way, it was hard to take some of the insults hurled at us.

When breakfast was over we begun preparing midday mess. I am sure we peeled a coal truck full of potatoes and as many onions. In the meanwhile the others were washing pots and pans. Several whole sides of beef were brought in for that mess. Fortunately there were men brought in to cut it, otherwise I'm afraid the poor steers would have been butchered all over again.

After midday, the evening mess preparations began immediately. I thought I would surely die from exhaustion before it was over. One friend of mine from Tuskegee, Alabama, who knew of my illness told me if he was in my position he would just collapse to the floor and be carried to bed. I did not do that because I felt I must, in fairness to myself, go as far as I could without giving up. I know now that my power of positive thinking was the only thing that brought me through that ordeal. The trip lasted three days and two nights. It seemed an eternity.

We arrived at Fort Leonard Wood, Missouri, at almost the same ungodly hour of the night as we were awakened at Fort Benning, Georgia, to come here. We were hurriedly unloaded and herded (not marched) into a clearing between double-deck barracks, assigned quarters then dismissed. I was badly in need of a hot shower but could not get within seventy-five feet of the showers, so many others had the same idea. They were stronger and were able to push forward. I took off my clothes and fell into bed on the lower of the double-deck bunk and was sound asleep when I heard someone yelling for me to get out of his bed. He was right, I was assigned the top bunk. I persuaded him to sleep up top tonight because I had gotten into his linen without a bath. We would exchange when we made our beds the next morning. My legs felt like they were transplanted from a long-time-dead cadaver, swollen but dead.

Fortunately the next day was squad orientation. I did not have to do much moving around. We sat around on the ground and listened to programs we were to follow when we began training. I was proud of myself for having weathered the first of many strenuous tests I was to go through in the immediate future. I wrote a short letter home telling about it and giving my new address.

The next day was Sunday, so I had a short reprieve from the pressing routine. It was not necessary for us to meet any roll call or even go to the mess hall. I stayed in bed until two P.M. I did not have an appetite for country-fried potatoes and sausage at the mess, so some friends and I went to the post exchange and ate ham sandwiches and drank Coke. We played the juke box so long until I knew the words to every song. We drank every soft drink in the PX, then went back to the barracks to play cards and shoot the breeze about what we would be doing if we were at home at this time Sunday afternoon. Playing cards for money was taboo so we only played whist or bridge for matches or whatever small objects we could use for currency. While everyone was involved in one game or another I gathered my toilet articles and went in to luxuriate in the shower. I stayed there so long I must have run the G.I. water bill over the limit for the day. I finally came out and climbed into my bunk for the best rest I had

had for almost two weeks. It was impossible to sleep, however, because of the din of noise around the card games. Lying there my mind drifted back home, to my family and what all this meant to me, to them and the people of the country, especially the south. In my estimation the coming of World War II ended an era in the South where cotton was king and black people were slaves to a vain hope of better things through its bounty. Two shots were fired in the South when that war began; one killed the poor sharecrop farmer and the other seriously wounded the big plantation owner's hopes of keeping him forever under his economic oppression. The phrase, "How are you going to keep 'em down on the farm," would come back to haunt those who visualized those young men marching back to the cottonfields. Many of them had been picking away at their dungeons of despair already; therefore being sent away to fight a war was for many a one-way ticket out of the South, out of reach of the white tentacle of oppression. I began to thank God for passing the physical. I realized that if I got nothing else but better medical attention I would be in better position to face whatever happened.

I knew that the rigorous military training ahead of me would be the supreme test of my endurance, both physically and mentally. I had to face it with all the determination I could muster, the time to separate boy from man being at hand for me. My resistance to sickle-cell attacks grew stronger as I learned more of what life was about. I was doubly determined not to live out my life in a nightmare of despair. I tried harder day by day to dispel the agony through mental power and spiritual acceptance. The training program began to move fast after a few days of instructions on basics. The drills were daily, the hikes longer and the personal equipment heavier. The obstacle courses seemed impregnable. The training became even more strenuous when a white major came out to speak to the troop assembly one morning. He began to cry as he spoke, complaining that the Japanese had destroyed Manila, some properties he owned there and killed some of his friends. He said, "I would love to go there and fight them with every damn thing I have but they need you worse than they do me; therefore I must remain here and see that you are ready to fight when you get there."

We were at the end of basic training and I was doing surprisingly well. My bones ached everyday, and only sheer determination kept me on my feet instead of flat on my back. I thanked God for the progress I had made and the ability to hang in there. I had been on sick call only two mornings during this time. They gave me some little white pills both times and sent me back to the company area. They were prone to labeling soldiers who went on sick call often, Gold Brickers. I think they gave everyone the same pills, whatever the complaint. One man from medics told us the pills were only unlabeled aspirin anyway.

I received a weekend pass and went to St. Louis to visit my brothers Lawrence and John. We had a great reunion. I had not seen them for many years. They lived in an apartment house, and there was a large restaurant downstairs where the cadet nurses from Homer Phillips Hospital gathered on Saturday evenings to have dinner. My nephew worked there, so when the girls came in he called to me to come down and meet them. Boy! This was a sight to behold. I had not seen a woman I was free to talk to in three months. They invited me to dine with them which I delighted in doing. During dinner and conversation I found they were invited to entertain soldiers at a U.S.O. Center that evening. I was invited to come along with them for the evening, as guest of all of them. They were well chaperoned at the dance but that did not prevent my making plans for a lone date early the next day.

Neither my brothers nor I had an automobile but fortunately the girl I picked for my date had one for that day. She came for me about noon on Sunday and took me on a short tour of St. Louis. We then drove to Forest Park Zoological Park—one of the largest in the country. I never knew places like this existed or that I would be allowed to enjoy it. We parked in a scenic area including a big blue water lake with flowers and water lilies. We sat there for hours talking, getting to know each other and watching the rest of that little corner of the world go by. It was mid-summer and days faded lazily away. We heard bird and animals calling in the distant zoo cages. The multicolored lights came on in the fountain on the lake. This should have been named Paradise Valley the scenic beauty of the flowers, trees and the lighted fountain spraying high into the dull evening light easily slipped us into a mood to seek a place of seclusion. I think it would be improper if not impossible to explain the pleasures we found in that seclusion. All I will say is that it was more wonderful than listening to the Duke play "Blue Velvet."

The night had fallen. Hot and humid in St. Louis, the hassle and trials I had in the last few months seemed far away and unimportant at that moment. The weekend had been most wonderful, but time was forcing me back to reality. I had to catch the bus back to Fort Leonard Wood and my date had to check into her dormitory by ten o'clock. She took me to the bus terminal. After the last good-by I boarded the bus and we waved until she faded out of my sight through the back windows.

On the road back to the fort as the big bus rumbled along I leaned back in my seat, closed my eyes and relived that weekend. I placed those few hours among some of the best of my young life. I did not write them in a diary but they are as vivid today as they were beautiful then. Riding through the Ozark Mountains with my window slightly open, the fragrance of the wild flowers was reminiscent of the wooded area at home. Suddenly the air brakes on the bus started wheezing and blowing, then the front door flew open and the driver called out, "All out for Fort Leonard Wood."

There were many other soldiers aboard. It was necessary for us to identify ourselves at the gate, name, rank and serial number. After passing though the gate I felt I had left something very important outside. It did not occur to me until I heard the trumpeter blowing retreat that it was my freedom I had left out there. The same old sauce was being served all over again; the drills, obstacle courses, and rifle ranges. We were to go on a thirty-mile hike in a few days, with full pack, battle gear, the works. I shuddered when I heard that news. It had been seldom that I rode that far and returned, much less walked. I had never invited a sickle cell attack deliberately, but it appeared someone else was doing it for me on a regular basis now. First the KP duty on that long troop train, the walking, running, climbing of training, now this big pin was aimed at my fragile balloon. There did not seem any alternative to going as far as I could, since I had reported ill several times with no attentions but those little white pills and a jeep ride back to the company area. Many times I didn't even get the jeep ride. The jeep was gone to pick up supplies on most of my visits.

The day of the long hike came quickly. No one was ready, I least of all. I knew this would be hell for me but felt I must shut that out of my mind and pretend I was as strong as anyone. The skies were overcast when the hike began, very pleasant for July in Missouri. After about four hours the sun came out. It seemed to beam down with vengeance because of having been held back by the clouds. We had been instructed not to drink a lot of water at once, but some of the men drank theirs as soon as the sun came out. Some became ill and had to be taken care of by the medical unit that followed us. Once I had learned to pace myself I did very well considering the circumstances and the fact I had outlasted some of the more vigorous men already.

We reached the half-way point just after noon. The kitchen had prepared chow, lamb stew, ugh. We were to have chow, rest about an hour and a half then start the return trip. Some of the men played baseball, some went swimming in a nearby lake, and others who were more exhausted by the walking sat or sprawled in the shade, hoping to have enough energy to get back to camp. That was my group who sat in the shade. I felt my muscles begin to tighten and my bones begin to ache, especially my legs and back. I approached the corporal of my platoon and told him I was not able to walk back. He took it very lightly. He asked did I want him to order my limousine or was I going to use a taxicab since I was out of town. He called me a goldbrick and said I would not get any sympathy from him.

The soldiers were soon called to assemble. I stood up and strapped my pack on. I had made only about ten steps toward the assembly grounds when my legs refused to go any farther. I fell forward, my face in the hot dust of the hills. I made no effort to get up. I knew I was fighting the monster again. I heard laughing from some of the men who thought as the corporal, that I was just trying to get out of walking back. No one there knew I would have given an arm and a leg to have been able to walk as far as anyone else. When they saw that I really could not get up some of the men helped me back to a grassy spot in the shade. The sergeant wrote my name and a number on a card and tied it on my pack. He told me to remain there. The medics would soon be there to pick me up to take me back to camp.

The sun was fading into the western horizon before the ambulance came for me, minutes had become hours, my pain increasing with every heartbeat. One of the men called to me to get a move on, and one said I could get up now that the others were all gone. When I told him I could not move he became a little more serious. The two men took the ambulance cot out and threw me on it as though I was a bag of fertilizer they hated to handle. The driver of the ambulance asked where he was suppose to take me, I said to the hospital, but the other attendant said he only had orders to take me back to the company area, the hospital was filled to capacity with sick men. I pleaded for medication for pain, but was told there was nothing they could do about that, they only picked up and delivered the men back to their respective companies. I was so exhausted, so I gave up asking for anything, and let them do as they wished. They had their orders and there wasn't anything I could say or do about that. I thought about his statement, "The hospital is filled to capacity with sick men." I felt that if there were any men there any more ill than I was at that moment, then he was already late for an appointment with his undertaker.

Final assembly and dinner were over when we arrived at my company. Men were milling around aimlessly in the area. When I was taken out of the ambulance, some laughed and said I should give it up, there was no way my act would convince the brass I was not just another gold brick. They did not know how near my act might be to my final curtain. I was taken in and thrown on my bunk, clothes, shoes, the whole works. I forced myself to get undressed and struggled into the shower. I leaned against the shower with water as hot and forceful as I could bear it. After about fifteen minutes I could stand without the support of the wall. I had left my clean garments in my locker at the foot of my bunk; therefore my struggle back to my bed in the nude must have been a bit comical to some who took nothing seriously.

Lockers were supposed to be kept neat but I only mustered enough strength to throw my things into it so that it would close. Then, with help, I climbed up on my top berth. Soon retreat was blown by the little trumpeter to signal the day's end. It was now time to rest from the toils of the day. I knew my toils were just beginning because I have never had an attack to go away without some kind of medical attention. I had none.

As the night progressed, so did the severity of my pain. I knew I was headed into the jaws of hell again. The blackness I had known so many times engulfed me minute by minute. I said all the prayers I knew and made up others. I used all of the mental strength I had through positive thinking. The hour was late and I had to hold on. *O God! please help, O God! please forgive if this is punishment. I am sorry for my sins.* I was not winning the battle, merely holding on. I had temporarily plugged the holes in the dikes of my sagging physical resistance with the fingers of my mind and prayers. Although the pain rushed through my body like a flooding Mississippi River, I did not cry aloud. I suffered in dead silence. Had I made a sound there at three A.M. I probably would have been hanged, because forty-nine other weary soldiers were sound asleep with the most important two hours ahead of them.

Finally the trumpet was sounding, sergeants screaming, men cursing, grumbling and getting ready for another day. I envied them all and would have traded for any task they might have had before them only asking to be able to do it without the awful pain that possessed me. Noticing I had not moved, the little corporal came back to my bunk, asking in a mocking tone, did I want him to bring my breakfast in on a tray or just send my valet in to dress me and take me out for breakfast. As I tried to explain he snatched the light covers off and shouted, "Get the hell out of that bed you stupid S.O.B., this is the army of the United States not a G.D. rest resort. You have five minutes, no it's three and a half now, now G.D it, let's get with it or I'll have you carried to the guard house flat on your ass on a stretcher since you enjoy lying down so much."

To avoid any conflict with him I made an effort to get out of bed. I convinced my legs to move over the side of the bunk. What I did not do was convince them they could hold me when they reached the floor, so I immediately collapsed to the floor in pure agony.

I think the corporal must have thought I was dead because I made no move after falling. He turned me over and put his head on my chest to see if my heart was still beating. Then he ran out calling for help. He called out to the sergeant. "Hey Sarge, I think this Crooms guy is dying. He fell out of bed and he's not moving. I think we should get him over to the hospital quick!" The sergeant came in and looked at me, he called my name several times but I did not answer him. He said to the other men with him, "I believe this guy is about gone, too, let's get him out of here fast. If he dies in here we might have trouble with some of the other men. We don't want that to happen to them before it's necessary they face death on their own when they go into battle somewhere, O boy!" His sympathetic thinking for the other men touched me deeply. I was dying and he was thinking of how someone else would feel if I did crumble there on that hard bare floor with not even a pillow under my head, having a chill by now because I was perspiring profusely when I fell.

The ambulance came, siren blasting, kicking up dust on the unfinished roads. The cot was brought in and when the attendants took one look at me and said, "Oh no, you mean this guy is dead again!" The sergeant said he thought it would be for sure very soon so get him out of here on the double. This was not the first time I had been counted among the dead, so it did not disturb me. What did disturb me greatly was the complete lack of humane feeling for a man that might really be dying or, but for the grace of God, would have been dead already. I did not want them to put on long faces or go into mourning but would have felt better with a slight touch of sincerity.

After my demise was discussed I was thrown onto the cot and taken to the hospital. I was placed in a private room (for VIP persons) and a quarantine sign on the door. I was in that room four days totally alone except an occasional visit from a doctor and a male attendant who brought me food and pills. The medication they gave me for pain was somewhat like a mosquito bite, including the itchy feeling around the needle. The doctors continually played the extent of my pain lightly. They thought it was an excuse I was using to get by without doing my duty. I am aware this is a hold statement, but most of the doctors there were very short on experience. They were young, proud of the gold and silver bars on their uniforms, but knew little about medicine.

This attack has lingered on longer than usual. I am not allowed to stand in the shower.

The shots for pain were discontinued after about eight days. The stiffness and soreness of flesh and bone were enough to make a mummy cringe. I was finally allowed out of my room in a wheelchair, I still could not walk. The attendant would sometimes take me to the back ramp of the hospital to sit in the mid-afternoon sun. The sun was warm and seemed to feed my body with soothing rays I needed very much. I felt blah, useless.

The *St. Louis Post Dispatch* was delivered to the various units on the fort. I read about the conflicts around the world; the Bataan death march, the Burma Road, Wake and the Solomon Islands were all far away, but had earth-shaking effects on the American people. I felt sad for the peoples of the world. Some were receiving extreme cruelty, others were inflicting it as though vengeance was theirs instead of only God's. Hitler was pillaging and murdering in Europe while I remember Tojo sought to make the whole South Pacific and Mainland America his imperial domain. Unlike our most recent Asian War, Hitler's murdering and Tojo's quest of imperial status over half of the world spurred young American men black and white into action that would ultimately right the wrongs of war.

I was finally sent back to my company area. Why back there I don't know; my company had been shipped out in preparation for overseas duty. I had mixed feelings about missing the boat, so to speak. I was placed in the quartermaster's unit dispensing clothing to new recruits. The freedom from the hospital did not last very long; I was called back for more tests. The blood tests they had taken earlier were confusing the people in the medical lab. They could not figure out why my blood cells were not round as others were. I was continually exposed to long sessions of questioning—who was your mother, your father, what did they look like, who were their ancestors, have you ever been ill like this before? I was even asked had any attempt ever been made to poison me? When all the prodding, poking and testing were over I was thoroughly exhausted. I was sent back to the same room, with the quarantine sign still on the door. I tried to remove the sign but was told to leave it. They thought I had some kind of malaria.

I am very tired now, I wish this was all over and I was free to rest or better than that—go home. It is late now, I cannot lie down.

I was restless so I sat down in my chair and placed my feet on the bed. I sat there in what seemed a twilight zone. I heard music and voices, but there was no one there. It was after ten P.M., therefore no one in the hospital wards was allowed to speak out or sing. I welcomed the music. It was a delightful contrast to the dismal suffering I was just emerging from. I do not know where the sounds came from, I leaned back and enjoyed them until it faded into the distance.

Despair was beginning to nag me now. I wondered where I would go from here. I couldn't imagine anything I could do in the service of my country as a soldier, so I wanted to go home. If I had to I was ready to say please, for I was weary in both body and spirit. I felt as though a vital part of my life's battle had been fought here in such short time. I was sorry to say I did not win. I gave it all I had but lost nonetheless. Although my heart was heavy and my steps slowed from stiffness caused by the sickle-cell anemia attack. I found no time for tears. I had to hang in there if I was to do anything with my life.

The course was mine along to chart. My family and old friends were hundreds of miles away and there were no personal counsels in the army. Everyone was on his own so far as personal decisions were concerned.

The attendant came for me early one morning for more blood tests. While I was in the medical complex the doctors had X rays made of my head. I never knew what that had to do with anything. I was taken back to my lonely room, ordered to bed and started receiving blood plasma in one arm and some other liquid immediately followed in the other. I have had more miserable days in my lifetime but it was long ago.

When the liquids were finished flowing into my veins, the evening meal was brought to me. The meal was one of my favorite dishes, ham, baked beans and a vegetable. I ate well but regretted quickly, as my stomach begun to boil like an over-heated teapot. In half an hour after I had eaten, everything that had gone down came back up, with some to spare. I began aching again, every fiber of me engulfed in pain. There were no bells or lights to summons help to it was necessary for me to call out to ask for help. I called out many times but no one came. I felt myself sinking back into the big volcano from which I had emerged just a few days ago. *Oh God! not again so soon, please help, dear God send me help, I don't want to die here.*

There was a glass vase on the table beside my bed that I knew would make a loud noise if I could reach it and crash it against the door. It took every ounce of strength I had but I managed to reach it and flung it towards the door as hard as I could. The vase landed with a loud crash, breaking into many pieces. In just a few seconds I had a room full of doctors, nurses, orderlies and some curious patients all wanting to know what had happened, why I threw the vase. When I told them I was very sick, they said I could have called to them, they were playing cards just across the hall. One of the doctors came over and began examining me, pinching my fingernails, stretching my eyelids wide, and poking his fist deep into my diaphragm area. He told the other doctors and nurses that the blood I had received earlier was definitely the right type but for some reason, unknown to him, was not compatable with mine. I had never had a blood transfusion before, therefore, the prospect of it having damaging effects was frightening.

My suffering had always been up to the brim of my cup but this difficulty with compatability of blood could be another spoonful added whether I could take it or not. I could feel myself losing strength. I began trying to hold back the onrushing tide of pain with my mind (thoughts) but to no avail. Everything came crashing in on me like an angered herd of bulls. I did not believe I would ever go as deep into the blackness of hell's caverns as I was then. I was surrounded by howls and screams. I smelled the stink of that ungodly place. *Oh God, please take me out of here. I am burning, I am tormented here, my life is on fire. Please, dear Jesus, ease my pains, ease my fears.*

This was the first time I had been given morphine intravenously. The young doctor treating me decided to give it to me after a long line of objections from the other doctors and nurses. He explained his reasons very simply, "Hell, he can't be any worse off than he is now. It might be a blessing for him if it kills him. If it brings him around he's out front, his pain is too deep for anything else to reach. It is worse than having a baby. I would rather have been at Bataan than where he is right now."

I too, would rather have been many other places I knew, preferably one of peace and rest without pain.

Soon I felt the prick of the needle and the medication entering my bloodstream. I could feel relief immediately. The morphine seemed to purge the pain, so after just a few seconds, the pain was dead and I was alive again even, if for a little while.

After an hour I drifted into the first real sleep I had had for many hours. I perspired heavily after morphine in-

jections so when I awakened the orderly was changing my
pajamas. When I was asked to sit in the chair so that the
bed could be changed I found my legs willing to obey orders to move me. While I sat in the chair I could feel some
pain still deep in my bones. My flesh struggled with heavi-
ness and seemed to be asleep. "If I could take a shower I
think the pelting of the hot water would wake it up." The
doctor vetoed the idea as soon as the request was made. He
felt I might faint after all the medications.

After several days I began feeling better. I sat in the
sun again and watched some WAC's play tennis. They
would not win any physical fitness awards but they were
graceful. They came over to talk for a while after having
finished their game. They asked me a thousand questions
about my physical condition. They asked many questions I
had no answers for. I wished they would go away, and finally they did.

I sat there until the sun was gone behind the big oak
trees of the Ozark Mountains, leaving purple-and red-
streaked clouds drifting about like lost sheep. I enjoyed the
quietness of the evening. The only sounds that disturbed
the stillness came from some energetic soldiers playing
baseball. I do not know how long I sat there, time is not
important when you have nothing to do anyway. My mind
went wandering, here, there, many places. I heard what
sounded like thunder but it was the sound of war. I saw
lightning but it was the fire that destroyed villages. I heard
voices, not in song, but in war chants. I heard music, but
iit was a call to assemble or to charge into battle. The
beauty of my dreams had faded into the bitter conflicts of
the world. I felt very much alone, although I was only a
few yards from hundreds of people.

As I turned to go, a beautiful girl stood in my path.
She was my friend from St. Louis. She said she had been
through the whole building trying to find me and was about
to give up and go home when a patient told her I was outside near the tennis court. She helped me up the ramp

with my wheelchair. She could see that I would never make it alone. We talked for a while before she told me she had come to say good-by for a while. She had been accepted in the Army Nursing Corps and had asked for overseas duty. It saddened me very much when she told me she doubted we would ever meet again. Before I could get my regrets out she was walking away. She turned at the end of the hall and waved back at me, walked out the door and I never saw her again. For me this was one more crash on a road already cluttered with accidents.

I am sure I was not alone, there were many final good-byes throughout the world so one more was not unusual. I did not know it at the time but I had said good-by to girl friends back home, some of whom I have never seen again to the present time.

The doctor was at my bedside early the next morning with papers for me to sign. He said I was on the list of nine to be given discharge. This made me very happy, except for one thing. I had not decided where I wanted to go, back home or to St. Louis. I had to weigh the potentials of both places carefully. I thought first of going home and back to school there, but had some misgivings because of the thought of never getting out of the deep South again. I had learned more about my chances there since I had been away than I had in all my life there. I couldn't see the forest for the trees. As I said before, not many Johnnies who were my friends would go marching back there.

I decided to go to St. Louis where my brothers Lawrence and John were living. I had not fully decided what I would do when I got there. I knew I must go back to school no matter where I chose to go. I knew nothing about the job market in St. Louis, nor the schools to attend when I arrived. After three days I was taken to the discharge center. I received two hundred and fifty dollars mustering out pay plus railroad fare back to Georgia. I bought a train ticket to St. Louis. I had called Lawrence and told him I would be there when I was released. I arrived in St. Louis in the early afternoon and took a cab to my brother's home on Eastern Avenue. They both lived in the same building. I felt as though I had fallen off an electric treadmill into a rocking chair.

After some weeks of relaxation my body was back in shape to move around freely. I was drawing military compensation but knew I must get a job because this would not last indefinitely. Through help from some friends I had met, I had started work at Liggett & Meyers Tobacco Co. The pay was so low they gave a carton of Chesterfield cigarettes with my pay every week. This is how I got started smoking. This job was hard work and soon proved to be more than I could handle. I went from small jobs to small jobs, attack after attack. There were many hours of discontent for me now. I was faced with so many things that led down hill. I finally passed the examination for a job at the St. Louis Ordinance Plant but only because I was a veteran and the doctor who examined me had a tendency to look the other way on things he thought were unimportant. This was the best one I had had since I had been here. Good pay and hours that would allow me to return to school. I learned the job well so I was elevated to inspector in a few months. I had never thought about having that much responsibility before. There were about thirty people I was responsible for.

The pace was fast at work and at school but I managed to adjust to both. Although things were difficult for me physically I managed to cope. There were many mornings when I had to think my way out of bed, along with lifting a leg out here and there. Not even my brother knew my problems of health, they only knew I kept on moving well between school and work.

Many of the people who worked along with me would help with my program when they found I did not feel well. I was always very grateful for that because they could have waited until I failed, then took the job for themselves.

I avoided a sickle-cell crisis for many months through positive thinking and fervent prayers. I did not blot it out, it is a chronic condition, but I did manage to slow its progress in destroying me. Compared to some of the other times I had in the past I considered these good times. The regular school year was over so I only had two hours in class. This gave me more time for rest, therefore, more strength for my job.

Everything went well for me until August of that year (1944). The day dawned hot and humid in St. Louis. I left for work at three P.M., wearing slacks and a very thin sport shirt. The weather was good when I entered the plant. Near ten P.M., two hours before time to go home, I saw lightning and heard thunder that shook the whole building. Rain came down in heavy torrents, whipped by the near tornado winds. When time for the shifts to change came it was necessary for everyone to clock out and leave the building. There was no place one could wait out of the rain until the bus came, therefore, everyone was soaked with rain and well whipped by the wind. I don't think I have been that wet even after a swim; the cold rain seemed to be beaten into my bones. When I reached home I felt as though I weighed four hundred pounds, every bone I have was stiff, my hands and face were numb. I did not have a shower so I got into a tub of hot water and wrapped hot towels around my head and shoulders trying to warm my body and possibly avoid an attack. I knew immediately that the hour's ride on the streetcar had been too long. The pain had started in my spine, arms and legs. I called the doctor, but he was an old man, therefore would not come out at that hour (2 A.M.). I got into bed and tried to fight back with my mind but could feel the darkness closing in on me. At five A.M. I was flooding down into the bottomless volcano, the heat, the dust and darkness had taken me out of reality. This is a horror chamber that could only have been conceived by the devil himself. After Lawrence saw that I was steadily getting worse he decided to take me to the hospital. My doctor finally came and gave me an injection for pain, the same flea flick I had received so many times before. It was not worth the walk he had just taken up three flights of steps. The doctor did serve a worthwhile purpose, however. He was instrumental in getting me a bed in the hospital, the trip that began my long history of hospitalization in different institutions in St. Louis, Missouri. I remember that trip so vividly because I think I had one of my worst attacks since I had been diagnosed.

I was exposed to modern medicine now but nobody seemed to know how to administer it at the proper time. My pain was so deep until the doctors feared I would become addicted if they gave me enough morphine to kill it. When I received one shot of pain killer, the way they gave it, the next four hours must pass before I received another became as an eternity in Hell's fire.

The nights and days were spent in agony. After eight days of exhausting physical and mental struggle I began to come out of the crisis. Although my body was numb I could command my facilities to work. I began walking from my ward bed to the therapy room where they had the only shower. The forceful pelting of the hot water helped to relax my stiff muscles.

The doctor who was attending me came in one afternoon to take a blood count specimen for the umpteenth time and starting discussing the kind of anemia I had, he ended the discussion with a question. "Do you know that people with this type of anemia don't live past thirty-five years?" I told him I had heard it before and would take the years he was giving me and ask God for many more. "I plan to live to age 81 and will invite you to my birthday party." I was released from the hospital four days before time to register for classes again. Lawrence threatened me with bodily harm if I went out of the house. He said there was nothing worth risking any further physical strain. I gave what he had said some thought but decided to register anyway. That was the most difficult streetcar ride I have ever taken, every bump of the old trolley shook every bone in my body.

I returned to work in early September and found that the arsenal was going on a limited operation. I was undaunted by this, it was one of many jobs I had lost. I had learned electrical welding earlier, therefore, was able to get a job with the Midart Manufacturing Company. I did not know the hazards of the job at the time, I only knew it paid more money than I had ever dreamed I would earn. They had a standard hourly wage piece work that paid well and all the overtime, holidays and Sundays I could make. There were two hazards; one was the density of the smoke and dust in the welding section of the not very well-ventilated, building. The other worst of the two, was the hot slag falling down from the welding rack and burning my jeans around my ankles. I found myself on fire many times. Blistering finally occurred around my ankles that would not heal. I went to several doctors before I found that I was susceptible to leg ulcers from the slightest aggravation because of sickle-cell anemia.

I learned to care for my wounds and continued to work everyday, many times seven days a week. I invented some buckskin leg shields that helped prevent setting myself on fire. As time went on the soreness of my legs became almost unbearable. The doctor recommended wearing ace bandages on both legs to take the pressure of the standing down to a bearable proportion. The bandages helped so far as the swelling was concerned but the pain was so great I often took three or four pain pills during the day, often two of any given dosage at one time. I endured this condition for more than a year. The only time I got back into any acceptable physical condition was when I went on vacation.

I spent the first ten days of that retreat from physical

woes in the hospital with my legs elevated under an in-fraray light that drew so hard on the excess fluids I had accumulated until it was necessary for me to have medication for pain. This stint in the hospital started my conversion to Catholicism. The nuns and brothers (Franciscan) were very pleasant and most helpful. I entered prayer and meditation every afternoon. The chaplain of the hospital came in to talk with me every day after prayers. We often said prayers alone, together. I enjoyed the closeness of all of them working there. This experience gave me more inner peace than I had ever known before.

I had a steady girlfriend, who came as often as she could to bring books and visit. We were to be married the next spring, at her Terre Haute, Indiana, home. She had just completed her R.N. program and was working at Homer G. Phillips Hospital (City Hospital #2).

When the ten days in the hospital were over my legs were still not completely healed. I asked the doctor to check me out anyway. I had planned to visit my parents for a few days of my remaining vacation. The doctor told me I would no doubt get sharp pains in my legs when I stood on them for the first time. What he did not know was that I had tried them many times before and would not be too concerned if they did not start bleeding as they had done before I came into the hospital. There were times, before I went to the hospital, when I soaked my feet after my bath that I felt traces of blood on the towel when I stepped out of the soak. I was still attending college; therefore, went to class many days so heavily sedated that it was necessary to take a wet handkerchief along to wipe my face periodically so that I could remain alert enough to do my work. The hours turned slowly into days, the days into endless time. Only determination kept me moving and the will of God alive. I have now learned to rely on both completely.

I packed my bags for my trip home that weekend.

There were so many bandages, salves, and other medications I hardly had enough space for other necessities. In those days blacks could not get Pullman accommodations from St. Louis south. St. Louis barely made it across the Mason and Dixon line. It was necessary for me to go all the way by day coach, about fourth class. Fifth class when I reached Knoxville, Tennessee, because the blacks had to move to the back of the coach to let the hillbilly farmers on with their produce and cages of chickens they were taking to market.

The war was over in Europe and Japan's knees were buckling under the devastating military forces of the United States but here in front of me was a shining example of, nothing has changed. Even though many black men and women had fought and died to save this country it was still necessary to sit in the back of the coach, still necessary for me to get sandwiches from the butcherboy instead of eating in the dining car, still necessary to go into the door that had a sign reading "Colored" when I came into a station. I was very tired from the long ride but refused to dwell on it. I sent my mind wondering over many other times passed. I had read the total contents of two *Reader's Digests*, and several newspapers.

The old slow train came into the station in Macon, Georgia, on schedule at one A.M. There was a six-hour stay there the train did not leave for Vidalia until seven-fifteen A.M. Those were six very trying hours. I could not relaxe any way I tried. Those seats in the station were as hard as Moslem slabs of marble and just as cold, the pot-belly stove had burned out, with no efforts made to revive it. My anxiety to see my folks had risen to a feverish peak by the time the train departed for Vidalia. My head and spine were throbbing like a toothache. I had only four hours in which to either pull myself together or go into another attack. There were only about sixty-five miles to go but the train stopped at every little pig path along the way, picking up dairy products, farmers with strawhats, old women wearing homemade bonnets and little boys wearing jeans worn out at the knees from shooting marbles.

There was a good number of empty seats in the back of the coach. I reversed the seat in front of me and put my feet up in order to keep down the swelling. I had hardly gotten comfortable before the redneck conductor came back and told me to remove my feet, that it wasn't allowed on his train. I placed my feet back on the floor, then took another dose of pain pills. The butcherboy came along with ham sandwiches and lemonade, I took a sandwich and two cups of lemonade. I drank one cup of the lemonade straight down then ate part of the sandwich. I sat there praying, "Oh God please give me this day, don't let my mother see me ill when I arrive home for the first time in over four years." I kept telling myself, "You must hold on, you must hold on." My mental facilities were hard pressed to convince my physical being to walk off of that train standing tall as my folks remembered me, but I managed to do it.

The only black cab in town was not at the station so I took my bag and walked the six or seven blocks home. I even ran the last block when I saw mother standing at the gate waving to me. I cannot express the joy I felt seeing them after so long a time. Mother said I looked tired and should go to bed and rest for a while before my friends found that I was home and started calling and coming to see me. I was in no condition to argue, it seemed the best idea I had heard. I had no rest since leaving St. Louis. The trip had been difficult. While mother fixed lunch, I took a hot bath and got ready for that heavenly bed. I had forgotten how comfortable those old beds were.

My mother fussing around the house, as she always had, brought back fond memories. Some of good times, some of bad. Dad seldom showed emotion but I could see the little glint in his eyes when he stood in the bedroom door talking to me. We talked about Lawrence and John and their families, how and what I had been doing. He wanted to know how my health had been since I had been away from home. I did not tell him the truth, I told him what he really wanted to hear—that I had been much better.

After having a hot bath most of the pain and tension was gone and I was able to sleep until half the afternoon was gone. I awoke to a lazy southern afternoon, children coming home from school noisily playing in the middle of the old clay street that passed our home. I also heard a few soap operas coming from people's radios in the surrounding homes, mother never listened to them, said she had more important things to do. I placed my feet on the floor and was surprised, in view of my near attack on the train, at the ease with which I could make them work. After wrapping on the yards of Ace bandages I dressed and went to the front porch to sit and talk with dad and watch the children go by. Some of them were younger brothers and sisters of some of the kids I had attended high school with. I had several visitors as soon as big brother and sister came home and had dinner. I saw the signs of changing times while they visited with me. First of all, some of those who came hardly passed the time of day with me in those years and their presence here said that we had now grown up and had more things in common to talk about. They asked many questions about where I had been, what I had done and was doing. Did I still have those strange spells come over me as I did while there in school? One of my high school girl friends stayed for dinner with me. In all this time some of those young people had not been out of the confines of Tombs County. They had been content to sit it out on a low back burner. I did not make them feel bad by saying I could not have done it. I had become disenchanted with Vidalia long before I was drafted into the service. I am sure, had I not gotten out of there I would have exploded or drowned in my own perspiration. I surely would have had my final attack long, long ago because the medical practice there was still as primitive as Abraham Lincoln's stovepipe hat. I knew this because mother told me her doctor told her she might be diabetic but did not affirm it any further or give her any diet or medication. Because I felt this poor medical situation still existed there I was very careful to take double supply of everything I needed to take care of myself properly.

Another girlfriend came by after a most sumptuous country fried chicken dinner prepared by mother. I am a compulsive eater when I feel like really getting into it so I packed it in to the very brim of my capacity. The girl and I then went riding, visiting some of the nearby farm families. Things were not the same with those people. The young men, just as I had thought, did not come marching back, they had sought greener pastures and families of their own and a new way of life that did not include wrestling the land in order to eat. My mind ran back over the years of back-breaking toil my folks had lived through on the farm, the joys, tears, and suffering, their refusal to complain. I closed my eyes and could hear my sister's and brothers' laughter. I felt the spirit of sharing what they had in those difficult years. They were nearly all gone from here now.

I remembered the revival meetings where my mother and father allowed themselves the luxury of shedding a tear, where they let the cares of the times fall away and reaffirm their faith that God would take care of you. Many of the things I thought of while my mind wondered over these years of illness had already come true. There were very few, if any, sharecroppers around any more. Very few young men my age came back to farm, or to Georgia for that matter. Black people had started a low-key resistance to white supremacy. Since the white landowners did not have the country side filled with "niggers" they were not as sure of their positions as before. After about four short visits to different places I was ready to return home, but my friend insisted I go to see her mother. The lady broke into tears when she found I was to be married soon. She said she always thought her daughter (who was driving me around) and I would get married some day. I am sure, however, I never gave her daughter that impression.

When we reached home my legs felt like elephant legs look. It was a struggle to make them get me out of the automobile and into the house without mother and dad realizing how lame I really was. Dad was elated with the Stetson hat I had brought him, but said I should not have spent all that money for it ($22.00). He was hesitant to wear it. Mother said she had never had perfume as nice as the vial of Evening in Paris. The way she had always came to my aid when I was ill I wish I could have given her the price of a sixty gallon drum full of it.

With all the people coming in so often and my going here and there I became very exhausted. I had to take a whole day and night out and stay in bed to get ready for my trip back to St. Louis. I was enjoying my visit but knew I must get back to work and school. My legs were in no condition to go anywhere but to the hospital. I knew this but no one else knew it, so I convinced myself I could do it if I tried. I tried and through the grace of God I made it work in my favor.

When I arrived back in St. Louis I moved into my own apartment on Vernon Avenue. The apartment was in a private home. I became friendly with the people there and lived as a member of the family.

It's Christmas now, and for the first time I can remember I do not have a Christmas tree or any decorations.

This was mainly due to my heavy schedules both at school and work. I was also having very serious trouble with my left leg, it now had dangerously deep ulcers on both sides and one on the shinbone. I almost shed tears every time I stepped off a deep curb or onto a streetcar. I took pain pills by the handfuls, with little relief. I had to cut my work schedule to five days with no overtime unless it was an emergency. Working under those circumstances really brought me down. I had to spend all the weekend, from Friday evening until Monday morning, flat on my back with my feet up, eating pain pills. Ms. Jones, my friend's mother, brought food up for me else I think I would have starved to death if my illness did not consume me first. She often pleaded with me to go to the hospital and remain there until my legs were healed, no matter how long it would take. She did not know those ulcers might take months to heal, if they should ever. I had to learn to live with them. I knew it would be as difficult as drowning Hell's fire with a garden hose but planned to try anyway.

Months passed before I was able to go out on dates or to a movie. I could seldom wear a proper dress shoe. This is why I do not like Hush Puppies. I wore them two sizes too large so many times. Winifred and I went out to the YMCA Annual "Y" Circus with some friends and were supposed to go to a cocktail party afterwards but I chose not to go because at a party of that type I was afraid of the agitation of getting around without some happy person stepping against my legs. We chose to stop at a small cafe and have a late snack then go to my place and play records or some games with the Robinsons. I ordered a french fried pork chop sandwich, she, an ice cream sundae. My chop was so tasty I ordered another. I did not feel I was overeating since I had not really had dinner, just a snack earlier. We sat there talking and playing our favorite tunes on the juke box, until I felt myself becoming ill. I knew this was a big one, my stomach was swollen, and seemed to have a dart contest going on with my spine as the dart board. Pains began shooting down both legs and arms. Win called a cab to take my home, all the cabs must have been gone to the "Y" Circus to pick up better fares than they could possibly get in the section of town where we were. It never came. I gave her a phone number of one of my friends and he came as fast as he could and took me home. I felt myself losing everything, the use of my arms, legs, even my eyes seemed dimmed from the severe pain down my spine.

Winifred called a doctor, and he, like the cabbie must have been looking for higher fees. He never came. She then called one of her doctor friends at the hospital. He lived in the neighborhood so he came immediately and examined me, then gave me a flea flicker shot. Fortunately, I had some fairly strong pain pills in my bedside table drawer to help the shot out a bit. When he was ready to leave Win went to show him out so I swallowed a pill dry while she was gone. I knew if she knew I would not have been allowed to take it along with the shot of pain killer.

In a few minutes, after the shot and pill, my heart began knocking in my chest as though it was trying to get out. Win called the doctor to ask what he gave me and found it was a small injection of morphine, very small, he said. She knew something had gone wrong so she began looking around for other medicine. She only had to go to the bedside table to know what had happened. She found the bottle of patent pain pills and asked me did I just take one of them. I admitted taking one because I thought the end of the road might be near. She began placing cold towels on my chest and neck. I thought that would surely kill me, but it only served to slow the strenuous heartbeat ing. Winifred called Lawrence and told him she had to be at work at seven in the morning. Lawrence told her to go on to work, take me with her and sign me in. He had to be at work at five A.M. and could not sign me in and make it back in time for his car pool to work. I was so miserable by five A.M. I had begun to wish I would pass out or become unconscious until something changed for the better. I was not so fortunate however. I began vomiting and having bowel movements at the same time. The food I threw up became green after about the third time around. I thought my stomach would come up any minute. There was no city ambulance service in St. Louis unless you were stabbed or run down by a truck, so it was necessary for Win to get a cab for us to go to the hospital. That was quite an accomplishment if you could pull it off at five o'clock on a Saturday morning. When the cab came there was no one but Win to get me downstairs and out to the sidewalk. Imagine, if you can, a 5'3", 117-pound girl trying to help a 6', 165-pound man who could barely stand up, down a flight of winding steps. The hedge along the curb seemed to move away as we approached it. The stupid cabbie saw that we were having a great deal of difficulty but sat there in the middle of Vernon Avenue and continued to honk his horn.

Fortunately I did not have to stop in the emergency room. One of Win's nurse friends who worked in receiving had managed to get a room for me, so with the use of a wheelchair we finally reached the room where I was to remain for nearly two months.

Our wedding was postponed for weeks. The doctors said that my gall bladder must be removed, so after a couple of weeks of coming back to the living we were married. Then I came back to the hospital for the operation. The doctors removed my gall bladder and planted the gall ducts directly into my stomach. Before the surgery I could not eat certain foods and there was always danger for me in eating late. I had had a stomach ache almost daily since I can remember. I found, after recovery from surgery, I could eat anything I wanted. I have become a pretty big eater since then. I eat anything, any time of day or night.

When I was well enough to leave the hospital I found that I was unemployed, the job had cut back to peacetime operations and I was working on a defense contract, that meant my hospital insurance was out also. Winifred, who was now my wife, said not to think of the bill, she would see that it was taken care of. I did not draw unemployment compensation because when I was able to get out and move about freely enough I got another job, without even making an application. My friend took me to work with him. He was friendly with the supervisor and there was no union to join before one could begin work. The job was difficult at the beginning but I suppose it was a process of becoming adjusted to things after such long time away from work.

During the doctor's exposition to find and remove my gall bladder everybody forgot about my sore legs. I think they must have decided to heal all by themselves because I do not remember having received any treatment for them. It was a pleasure to get up in the morning without wrapping in the yards of Ace bandages.

During my most recent illness I lost thirty pounds so my doctor had put me on a high fat, high sugar diet to bring my weight back. I gorged every day with all that rich food. Chocolate cake and candies were my favorite. Many times I have eaten a double layer box of candy in a single day. Win had many friends among the doctors and nurses at the hospital who remembered me and often sent me boxes of candy. I suppose people, including doctors especially, have always had a vicious streak that shows up now and then. Winifred came home crying one afternoon because one young intern asked her why she married a dead man. He thought that I would surely be dead within two or three years at the most. I told her to put that out of her mind, I had many things I planned to do before I decided to leave this earth and they could never be completed in the two or three years this young know-it-all had given me. One other thing, I did not believe he had been given any years to split up between anybody; therefore, his prediction failed to disturb me.

I had been advised to change my course at school. My school finance was running out and I did not have enough hours to get what I was seeking in that field. I entered the St. Louis College of Mortuary Science in September of 1946. I went into this with much determination. I knew this was a one-way street. I place emphasis on this because working in the factory had become increasingly difficult. I knew I could not continue this type of work for much longer; my legs broke down at the slightest provocation. In the department where I was working, my hands and arms became so soaked with oil and grime that it was necessary to do the family wash to get them clean enough to go to church on Sunday. I continued to have threatening attacks frequently. I was able to avoid going all the way down with some of them, Win was a very trusted and efficient registered nurse, so was allowed to keep a more potent pain medication than the doctor would give directly to me.

My job at the factory had to be abandoned after I began mortuary school, classes were held during the day and my job was a day shift also. I did not have many regrets. It was becoming too strenuous for me to attend school and work a full-time job anyway. I got a few hours per night cleaning a furniture store to supplement my G.I. school program. This gave me more time to concentrate on my studies. The school program posed little problems for me; I had already had a number of hours credit in anatomy, bacteriology, and microbiology, three of the major subjects. I faced one problem however; the hesitation of some of the funeral directors to give me an apprenticeship. Some of them wanted me to pay them a certain fee besides working full time. I finally was accepted by the C.T. Nash Funeral Home in East St. Louis, Illinois, for a salary of twenty-five dollars a week and a room in their home over the funeral parlor. I suppose this was the generally accepted thing for an apprentice. I did a little of everything. Cleaned cars, hearse, swept the sidewalk, fed the dog, cleaned up behind him, took him out walking and a little of the embalming. The most trying of my duties was going along as an ambulance attendant. It was a private ambulance but we picked up every kind of case from auto accidents to women having babies, many of the women having the babies called too late. I'm sure I helped deliver at least five on the way across the McArthur Bridge to St. Mary Infirmary in St. Louis. Two or three calls a night on the weekend were not unusual, rain or shine, sleet or snowstorm. I often became so exhausted until I wished I could just get on the ambulance cot and tell the driver to take me to the nearest hospital and leave me until I called him about a month later to come back for me. I had many, many restless nights from soreness and stiffness in my back and extremities because of lifting ambulance patients and dead bodies twice my weight down two and three flights of steps and into the hospital bed or onto the preparation table. Many of the deceased ones I embalmed before I was able to get back to bed. This continued for a year, with time out for some disabling attacks and many overnight or weekend near misses.

When I had passed the Illinois embalming examination the owner told me he did not have a job for me as a licensed embalmer and funeral director but offered me a job carrying a debit for an insurance company in which he was part owner (burial insurance). The insurance debit was scattered all over East St. Louis; therefore entailed a lot of walking since I did not own my own automobile. I took the job for what I thought would be a few weeks but the weeks turned into a year. I walked many miles daily through the streets of East St. Louis and Brooklyn, Illinois, and the "Hill," the stockyard area. When the wind was high, as it often was up in Brooklyn, the dust was blinding; when the rain came, this dust was ankle deep slush that got into my shoes and irritated my legs, making every step there dreaded. When I visited the stockyard area on a windy day, the stink, mud and flies were unbearable.

Near the end of that year I passed the Board of Mortuary Science in the state of Missouri. I made several applications to funeral homes in St. Louis and was accepted by the E.B. Koonce Mortuary Inc. The wages were low and the hours long but there was more dignity and much less walking. The job also offered a future in my field. This was a beginning of the fulfillment of the goal I had sought for many years, to have a profession instead of a job in a factory or other places where every day was a test of my physical strength. My early years in this position were some of my best up to that stage of my life. I had moved back to St. Louis and had a company car at my disposal. There was only one catch in having a company car, it was necessary to get up any time of night to make a first call for the funeral home. I caught many colds that way because since childhood I have always perspired during the night, and the way the business came in St. Louis, any call we received was an emergency. That left me little time to get myself ready for a winter night outside. During winter months I sometimes went to the doctor two or three times a month to combat colds. A chest cold can trigger a sickle cell attack quicker than anything I know. The pain begins in the rib cage and spreads rapidly over the entire body. This is maddening pain. The diaphragm seems to tighten so that the thoracic cavity is almost paralyzed. There is also pressure on the whole abdominal cavity and during times like that, I could not eat if my life depended on it. If food went down at all, it came back immediately. As time wore on I had more responsibilities added. Funeral services were held at night in St. Louis and this meant long days for everyone especially the director. Many times I came to work at seven-thirty in the morning and worked until eleven at night. The ulcerations returned to my ankle and lower legs, sometimes worse than before because I was not allowed the luxury of wearing just any old shoes. I had to look sharp every day. I had a variety of duties now, supervisor of the chauffeurs, directors, and secretaries, meeting people and arranging funeral services. I think I must have grown a fixed smile on my face during that time so that I would not succumb to the terrific desire I often had to grimace because of the pain in my legs, often everywhere else.

Trying to walk on the sore legs often created nagging back aches I would not otherwise have had. There were very few times when I could just sit in my office and prop my feet up and relax, there was always something to do or supervise.

My father died in October, at my home in Georgia. My wife and I took the train down for the services, also to help with funeral arrangements. Since I was then a director I had some different ideas as to how I wanted things done.

This was a taxing trip, just as the one I had taken to visit a few years before. I had the same problem, I was thoroughly exhausted and had the same sore legs. One thing was in my favor, however. Winifred was with me with better medication than I had the first time.

We were not allowed a Pullman this time either. Leaving St. Louis was still leaving the South headed south, so this was the same old straight-back seated coach all the way; the same six or seven hours on the morgue slab seats in Macon. The fire was burning in the pot-bellied stove this time, even in the "Colored" side, but the heavy coal smoke was escaping through the burnt pipes before it reached the exit. It became nauseating to the point everyone had to go outside in order to breathe. I had eaten a lunch Win had brought with her and the smoke almost made me part with it. The police came by on his patrol of the station and ordered everybody back into the building. Fortunately it was almost time for the train to arrive, so we walked back into the smoky room just long enough to get our belongings and go out to the boarding platform.

We were on our way home very soon. I was enjoying a small relief from my leg pains, but the weariness of the rest of my body lingered. I wanted to get into a tub of hot water so badly I could almost see the tub before me.

After arriving home and relaxing some of my brothers and I went to the funeral home to complete financial arrangements and view our father's body so that the larger number of people could be allowed to come in to view him. There were no emotional outbursts there. I do not think the full impact of his death had hit us. The funeral service was to be held the next afternoon at the Hopewell Baptist Church, where he had been on the deacons' board for nearly forty years. The little white church sat up on a hill in a vacant field. I did not really get the message dad was gone until the bell began to chime and his old friends came by to say words of encouragement. He died at age seventy-six from a cancer he refused operation for. He said,

"What God has put together let not man disturb, this is his will therefore mine also. I will die with what he has given me to die with." Some considered this ignorance of modern medicine, I considered it raw courage.

My older brothers were the pallbearers. I wanted to be one but my physical condition had prevented me, as it had so many times, from being as normal as the others. After having obtained funeral director's license and working with emotional people I thought I could handle my dad's death, but the feeling is very different when the deceased is someone you love. I refrained from outward emotions but inside I could feel something tearing at me. I felt my rib cage becoming tight; my arms and legs seemed to be dead. I could not leave the car for the graveside services. I just sat there staring into space, thinking about my father, some of the difficulties he had lived through. I never saw his head bowed except in prayer; I never saw him walk around obstacles, he always managed to walk over them; I never heard him express regrets, he had so many mouths to feed, he always managed to feed them. I do not think he had an enemy in the county. They all stood around the grave that afternoon, some in their best suits, some in overalls, all with heads bowed to hear the last prayer—to say the last good-by to their old friend. There was no trumpet to play taps, no drums to roll or organs to play, the meaning of good-by came through loud and clear on that chilly afternoon when the senior choir burst into song: "I Ain't Got Long to Stay Here," then "Jesus Keep Me Near the Cross." The emotions I felt then, along with the deep-seated pain in my body, was much too much for me. I returned to the family home immediately and got into bed where I remained for most of the next two days. During that time I was in mortal combat with sickle-cell anemia. There was no hospital nearer than Macon, where my father had just died a few days ago. I knew I had to win that battle and get back to St. Louis to doctors who knew what was happening with me. It took everything I had but for once I was the victor.

Mom asked Win to take care of me; she was leaving me in the hands of the Lord; she had gone as far as she could and would soon be going where dad was.

The trip back to St. Louis was long and silent. We did not talk about my father's death. Win was afraid it might upset me again. A few days after my wife and I arrived back in St. Louis my very best friend, Dr. Elizabeth Courtney, died. I had been host in her office receiving her patients evenings after school. It was during this time she exacted a promise from me to take care of her when she died. I regretted that promise a million times since time had come to fulfill it. The effects of my father's death and the grueling pace I had kept in recent weeks were still leaning heavily on me. I had sharp pains throughout my body, alternating every day, and the recent emotional pressures I had experienced were pushing me to the breaking point. Mentally I felt my world caving in, physically my body. I summoned all the strength and courage I had for those few days my friend was lying in state. The constant flow of her friends, patients, and well-wishers kept the funeral parlor open nearly sixteen hours a day. I was there on my feet most of them. My whole body ached as though I had been beaten with a blunt instrument. When the services were over my body was ready for hospitalization but I was fortunate enough to have a weekend off so managed to recuperate enough to keep going. I must have gotten under the shower at least ten times during that weekend, trying to soothe my sore muscles.

In less than ninety days from my friend, Doctor Courtney, my mother died at our home in Georgia. Along with my brother Lawrence and his wife, my wife and I started out on that same train home. The snow began to fall as we were leaving St. Louis and by the time we reached Tennessee it was coming down in blizzard proportions. When we had reached the middle of the Tennessee mountains the heating system of the train went out of order and finally the whole engine. We were stranded in the middle of nowhere in several inches of snow with no heat, in a passenger coach that already had frozen mist on the inside of the windows even before the heat went off. Lawrence bought a bottle of whiskey from the porter and paid him to get some blankets to wrap around us. I took a drink of the whiskey, the first in my life, to get warm. That one drink of whiskey taught me that alcoholic beverages are deadly to one who has sickle-cell anemia. My heartbeat was accelerated to a very high pitch in just a few minutes. I began to perspire so profusely until I was forced to remove the blanket. I became chilled almost immediately and along with the chill came the pain. The veins on the back of my hands and in my temples became distended almost to the bursting point. I know now, that they were the same wherever they were located, those were only the ones we could see. I wished I could become mercifully unconscious but knew from past experiences this would not happen. People with sickle-cell anemia always remain conscious enough to feel every stabbing pain. It was necessary for me to endure this pain for about three hours before my wife thought my pulse rate had subsided to the point where the pills would not be dangerous. I am glad she thought of that because with the severity of the pain I had, I probably would have taken a double dose.

We were stranded there approximately five and a half hours until another engine came from Memphis. I can never explain why I did not have a full-fledged crisis. Once the train was warmed and on the way again I actually felt better than I did when we started the trip.

Charley came to Macon to pick us up, since the train was so late. We would not have gotten a train home until the next day. We were too late for the last train and much too early for the next.

The death of mother was harder for me to take than dad, not because I loved him less, but because this was my mother, my nurse, my strongest ally and my mediator to God long before I could speak for myself. She had done everything for me one person could do for another, yet she asked nothing of me. She had rocked me on her knees all through the night, then prepared meals all day for everyone along with many other chores of the day.

I was sitting again where I had sat such a short time before. I listened to some of the same hymns. The Rev. Salomon was saying some of the same words, reading the same Scriptures he read for my father. Special songs rang out from the choir loft. "Steal Away to Jesus." The old church seemed to sway to the rhythm the low sweet humming from the deaconess's corner would have penetrated the hardest shield of armor in the world. I do not think there were many dry eyes there that afternoon. I tried hard to control my emotions but my tears were perpetual. I wondered, while standing in our small family plot, was there a reward great enough for her? She had given so much to have had so little, yet she often sang because she was happy and smiled when there could have been tears. I shall never forget that afternoon for two reasons: first, I was bidding a last farewell to the best friend I ever had, and secondly, this was my thirtieth birthday.

Some of my brothers walked from the cemetery to the family home. This was a short distance, but I dared not try it, I felt all used up—numb. My feet and legs were swollen but not too painful for the moment. I had been heavily sedated since we arrived here so I suppose you could say I was saturated with pain pills.

The trip back to St. Louis was uneventful. The incident of the stalled train in the snowstorm taught me to always take a blanket along thereafter. When I went back to work at the funeral home every service reminded me of my mother and father and my friend. I cried a million tears during those next few months. My heart was heavy and my body was becoming heavier every day. My left leg became progressively worse until I had phlebitis up to the knee. I would wrap it in the morning and by noon the bandages would be soaked through and sticking to my trouser leg.

My temperature was very high. I was just plain sick, not ill, sick, sick, sick. I knew hospitalization was inevitable. I drove myself to the doctor's office and he took one look at me and said: "Give me your keys, I'll call your office and have your car picked up. You will be going to the hospital from here in the ambulance." He brought me into his treatment room and split my trouser leg to a few inches above my knee. His congenial conversation ended when he took that soggy bandage off and looked at my leg. He exclaimed in disbelief at what he saw. He walked away with his hand to his forehead and called back to me, "Why in hell did you let that leg get out of hand. We might have to remove your leg, man. I just will be damned."

Ours was not just a doctor-patient relationship, we were longtime friends. I could feel myself losing ground while lying there on the table. My heartbeat seemed to be sending out sharp bits of hot steel instead of the blood it was pumping. My blood count was so low the doctor hastily ordered blood to be available at the hospital when I was admitted. I protested against receiving blood, I remembered what had happened when I was transfused while in the army hospital. The doctor won the battle and transfused me anyway. For the present the blood transfusion seem to have worked. I was able to sit in a wheelchair with my leg elevated and move about the hospital and talk to my friends. All of the people there knew me by now, I had been there so often. The sun was warm that day so I rolled my chair out to a little balcony on my floor and played checkers with an older man who was a frequent visitor in the hospital also. Soon the nurse came out with medication and rolled me to my room for a rest period. I was only in bed a short time before I felt nagging pains in my spine and pelvic bones. I pulled my bedside light on to call the nurse. She came and I asked her to call the doctor. By the time the doctor arrived the pains were unbearable. I screamed as I had never done since I became an adult.

For the first time I can remember I was allowed the

mercy of unconsciousness. My wife told me later they had called her at her work and advised her to come to the hospital immediately if she wished to see me alive. Several doctors other than my own examined me and informed Win they did not find any cause for my condition but doubted I would last (live) until morning. I did not know until three days later that for all intents and purposes I was dead. I had a long history of coming back in spite of the doctor's prediction, so I defied the doctors and the grim reaper again.

When I was able to recognize things I found I had tubes everywhere they could stick one in. This was a very slow recovery. I had to learn to walk again. The hospital evidently did not have a therapy lab available this time because my push for recovery was done solely by one. The only medication for my particular case was antibiotics and pain pills. I took the pain pills nonstop for more than two months. Many times after taking pills the pain was unbearable before time for the next dose that should have been taken. I read every book and magazine I could get to try and keep my mind elevated above my health problem. I had been away from work so long I did not really know whether I still had a job. The nagging aches and pains seemed to be endless so I decided I might as well suffer them in my own home where the bed was softer and the food more palatable. I signed myself out of the hospital and took a taxi home. Winifred was still asleep when I opened the door to our apartment. She sat up in bed as though she was looking at something unpleasant from the past. She said, "You are going to be the death of me yet. What are you doing home?" I explained I might as well be at home. I could eat pain pills anywhere, and that I would rather eat them at home.

I remained at home about ten days then returned to work. I was grateful to find I still had a position with the company. I have lost many jobs because of long illnesses like I had this time. Nothing had changed at work, the pace was still fast. I was spared some duties until I was stronger. There was no way for me to regain any of the salary I had lost; therefore, I had some very lean days financially. My wife was working but I did not know where her earnings went. I did not know what she earned until I filed her income tax; therefore, I had two problems, each aggravated the other.

I learned from this to do my very best with what I had and thank God for it. I have been fortunate to some degree, I have never been without a job when able to work on one, nor have any unusual or undue concessions been made to me because I was ill. I was soon going full stride at the mortuary again. I worked very hard to perfect my skill as a mortician, and was soon considered by many as one of the best in the state. This enhanced my position with the company, it also helped to lift me out of my financial dilemma. Over the next two and a half years I considered myself very fortunate, although I was constantly nagged with the discomforts of sickle-cell anemia. I did not have a full attack, that is, one that hospitalized me.

I came into my office one morning and asked were there any calls during the night. The secretary gave me the call sheet and I saw that we had a soldier shipped in from California. I took the pouch from the clipboard and opened it to check the death certificate. I looked at the cause of death and it seemed to jump out at me. This young man was only twenty-two years old and the death certificate read, *cause of death: sickle-cell anemia—contributing cause: infected ulcerations of both legs.* My spirits sank to the level of my feet—flat on the floor. My mind went back to the time I was in the service, the difficulties of that time in my life. I could hear the secretary calling my name, asking, "Are you all right, Mr. Crooms? What's wrong?" She seemed to be miles away instead of sitting right in front of me. I finally snapped back to the present. I know it was only a minute or two but it seemed like years since I opened that envelope. I said a silent prayer for the young man back there in that casket. I did not notice how long he had been in the service, nor how he could have gotten there as modern as medical science is today, almost fifteen years since I was there. I wondered was his physical hell the same as mine, and did he also go into the bottomless volcanoes, as I had gone, over his short years on this earth? Had he walked in the valley of the shadow of death as I had walked, and was still walking at the old age of thirty-five— twenty years more than any doctor gave me to live?

The family came into my office to complete burial arrangements. I talked with them at length and found they never knew what his condition was, what or why he had been seriously ill all his life. I did not try to explain to them, not being a doctor; I felt I might mislead them and compound their grief. This disturbed me for many days. I had been told so many times I would not live past twelve, then nineteen, then twenty-five; I was thirty-five waiting for some young doctor to tell me I could not live to thirty-six.

It seemed to be a farce when the lieutenants, colonels and regular army men came to give him a military service. I suppose this was just the way I felt, the family thought he was properly honored. The sound of the trumpet was the sad tune I had heard many years ago, the firing of the salute was like thunder, frightening everyone there who was not acquainted to the procedure of military burial. If the pageantry there that day had been channeled into medical research they might have found something to combat sickle-cell anemia, or at least make a start. I wept as much as any member of the family, my tears did not come from my eyes they came from my soul. I wondered how many men buried beneath those endless columns of white stones had died this way without their families knowing why, without the military authorities ever caring. I am sure there must have been a good number of them, like many other people with various diseases. Sickle-cell anemia has been hidden under a bushel basket, nothing was done until very recently.

The emotions I felt while standing there in the Jefferson Barracks National Cemetery, on the banks of the Mississippi, were enough to send me directly to the hospital. I knew my condition had been named (sickle-cell anemia) but there must be something more to it then just a medical term (not a disease). No matter how I tried I never won decisively whatever my task, sickle cell seems to persist enough to spoil things, or at least let me know it was there waiting to engulf me if I gave the slightest indication I was ready to give up and be a run-of-the-mill invalid. I must admit I have given thought to concession, but I had learned how disastrous this would be for me, my family and friends. Too much of my blood and tears had gone over the bridge. I had conquered so many fears, grabbed a reasonable education and qualified myself for one of the better positions in my field at the time. There was too much to lose, it took so much to gain it. There was never relaxation from push and concern, whatever I was about my peace is like a morning cloud, like the dew that goes early away. (Hosea 64.)

No one knew the height of my emotions at this stage of my life. I think emotional strain now caused me more discomfort than anything else.

The rapid pace I had to keep at work, the ordeal of some of the boring social functions I had to attend and the steadily growing disagreements between my wife and I were like three slabs of lead placed on one side of a scale of justice against cotton balls on the other. I knew I must do something to balance the scale as quickly as possible, else the consequence would be grave. My nerves were like jagged pieces of glass; I had headaches when I got out of bed every morning and when I returned to bed at night. This was compounded by the fact I could not let this be known by letting myself go. I held a high position at my place of employment. I could not deal with the other employees with a bad attitude which continuous headaches created. I asked no quarter during this time. I was often complimented on doing a fine job on this or that project. I have often taken care of three funeral services in one evening without anyone knowing how ill I was. A bottle of pain pills did not last very long; I literally ate them all day and most of the night. I did not sleep well and could not take sleeping tablets because my heart was already so hard pressed by the pain pills that it often had an irregular beat—out of normal rhythm. Meanwhile, the differences between Winifred and I finally came to the point of no reconciliation. We began divorce procedures in October. The divorce took almost two years. Winifred became so abusive and antagonistic towards me until it was necessary to have the secretaries screen the calls to my office. I had a business phone from my office installed in my apartment; therefore, I did not answer my private phone at home for many months. During those months I had many aggravating attacks. I seldom went out except for work. The constant bickering back and forth between lawyers and clients was enough to send me to Arsonal Street—the mental institution in St. Louis. It was finally over and I was broke, cleaned out of everything she had asked for, savings, furniture, the apartment, even my insurance policies. After all of that she came to the parking area and took my new automobile and kept it for three months—until the finance company repossessed it. Then I had to buy my own car back from the finance company.

When this was over I had a four-day attack that seemed a year long. I had pains in my neck and shoulder so severe I could hardly see across the street. I often shook like a man with palsy, my whole system near a collapse and my doctor powerless and my power of positive thinking was just a phrase. Just as swiftly as that attack took me down I was up again. I knew only God could have done that.

There are many more ordeals that occurred during those two years getting a divorce but they are too personal, irrelevant and probably would be boring. Financial difficulties beset me again after the divorce, all my savings were gone into my ex-wife's bank, lawyer fees and doctor bills. I went into the city hospital with my next attack, the first time, through necessity, in my life. As I have stated before, I have never received any financial assistance from anyone, nor have I ever asked for any. I have spent enough on medical bills during my lifetime to be a wealthy man, if I could have saved that amount.

The same body pains plagued me daily, not completely putting me out of action but often impeding my progress so that I felt I would lose my determination to go on. There is always fear of stagnation if I give just an inch in this constant battle. I met a very fine young woman; Mari Stoncil, who came to the funeral home to work during her vacation from college. We became very close friends, so close, in fact, we were married about a year later. Our love and the fun we had together boosted my mental attitude out of the darkness it had been in for many years.

I still had physical difficulties but I had a good mental attitude to fight with. After some months my wife became pregnant; our happiness had her on a high plateau. After about seven months of this happiness I noticed my left leg began to swell from the knee down. The soreness in my leg and foot became almost unbearable, so much so that I began using a cane to keep some of the pressure off of it. In a short time I had ulcers on both sides at the ankle. I received antibiotics from my doctor often but the ulcers continued to grow larger. Every time I wrapped my leg in the morning there was a little more space to cover and a little more pain to prove it was getting worse daily. It became so sore and raw that I had to arrange my time so that I could sleep, when I was relieved enough to sleep, with my leg uncovered because the cover irritated the sore areas. My doctor refused to put a permanent bandage on for fear the seepage would irritate other parts of my leg it might touch, although, wearing the bandage all day at work did that anyway.

Mari was nearing her time to give birth and I was

nearing a hospital ward myself. Three weeks before the baby was to be born my doctor demanded I get off of my leg. He checked me into the hospital and began treatments on my leg, and also treid to prevent this from throwing me into a sickle-cell anemia crisis. A consulting physician told me that I had phlebitis in my leg and he thought it might have to be amputated if the treatments I were receiving did not work quickly.

I cried out, *Oh Lord, please don't let this happen, I have taken everything that has been piled on me all these years.*

I think I must have said prayers non-stop for the next three or four days. I had more to hang on for than I had ever had before, a very loving and understanding wife and a baby coming very soon. I say to you that I have never felt that way before. If that leg was amputated I did not see how I could possibly go on. I already had a split hip joint that crucified my right side, so this probably would put me on crutches for the rest of my life. If every prayer and pleading I said in the days that followed had been written I am sure you would have had a ten-inch volume.

To everyone's surprise my leg began to get better, and although I came right to the very edge, I did not go into a crisis. My wife came to see me often. She was so heavily pregnant I became afraid for her to come. She came to see me on Saturday afternoon, February 13, and we had a long happy visit. When she was ready to leave she said, "Bye darling, the next time I see you we will have our little baby girl." The next morning my friend, who had brought her to see me came to the hospital and told me he had taken her to St. Marys Hospital during the night and that our baby girl was born at 8 A.M. Sunday morning just as she had said it would be.

This was a Valentine's Day and the baby's birthday. I knew I must see her so I called my doctor to ask if I could

*be released from the hospital so that I could go to my wife
and baby.*

The doctor said I could not go because my leg was still
not healed. I went to the nurse's station and asked for my
leg to be dressed immediately so that I could put an Ace
bandage on it, that I was leaving the hospital. She looked at
me with a shocked expression on her face but sent a nurse
in to do the dressing. My friend took me to a florist and gift
shop near the hospital where she had delivered. I bought a
dozen red roses and a beautiful heart-shaped box of candy
and took them for her. There was no visiting hours at that
time of the morning; therefore, I had to explain for fifteen
minutes before I was allowed on the maternity floor. Mari
was still somewhat groggy from the ordeal, but wanted to
know how the baby looked. I told her she would have to
see her to believe how pretty she was, an angel with a
rosebud mouth. I visited with her for a short while then returned to the (my) hospital.

I was checked back in for three days, then released in
time to bring my wife and baby home. After about seven
days at home with my new family, I took my usual hot bath
that night before bed time and carelessly slept with my
shoulders out from under the cover. When I awoke the
next morning I could not move my body out of bed. I felt
as though I had become paralyzed, I was so stiff and sore I
could neither pull the cover up or push it down if someone
else placed it. Mari called the doctor and he was in one of
those he's-going-to-die-anyway moods, so he did not come
right away. He sent some pain pills through the pharmacy
delivery service. I thought he had forgotten he had the pills
and gone home. When the delivery man finally arrived, the
on-rushing tide of pain was deeply rooted in my body so I
might as well have been taking aspirin one at a time.

I ate that evening, Mari called the doctor again and informed him that I was getting worse. He came after his
office hours were over—about 9:30 P.M. He seemed irritated
when he came in, he gave me a strong injection then sat

down to discuss my condition with my wife. He began by telling what I had heard a thousand times already. "Ms. Crooms you will have to get used to seeing him like this, he might get better this time but he can't live much longer. It's impossible, he has already lived past the general life span of a person with sickle-cell anemia." He did not realize that I was lucid enough to understand in spite of the heavy injection. I vowed then to outlive him. He died about 1961, still a young man. I have buried many doctors that way—those who predicted a short life for me. (I take no pleasure from this.)

I was determined to get better as quickly as possible, we were still living in my bachelor's apartment. There was not enough space for the baby's bed to be set up; therefore, she was sleeping in the dresser drawer and when we needed the couch for sitting, there wasn't a resting place for anyone. Mari had furniture but we must first find a suitable house to put it into. Another reason we must get out of this apartment, is that my wife must walk down three flights of steps just to get the mail or send a letter.

After many days of struggle and a couple of bottles of pain pills I finally shuffled out to work, over my doctor's objections. There have been very few times in my life that I have been released by my doctor to return to school, to work or any other place after a severe attack, I have always had to make that decision myself because only I knew how I felt. No one could know unless he or she had sickle-cell anemia.

If pain was material each person who has sickle-cell anemia would have created a mountain that would challenge Mt. Everest in magnitude. Only thirty years of life is 10,950 days and as many nights of suffering our days are longer than usual. If every prayer I have prayed for peace of body was recorded the volume would be endless. Even while working at a full-time job I said prayers long and sincerely before I allowed myself to take a pain pill. My wife often told me I looked like some kind of nut walking around in pain and would not take the pills I had in my pocket. I often avoided taking them that way.

The pain did not go away. I forced myself to live with if for longer periods of time. I believe this has helped my heart to last longer and maintain better condition. Mari and I found a suitable apartment, furnished, and moved into it. She then took the baby and went to visit her mother in Ashland, Kentucky. The food she prepared for me before she left was soon eaten. Working all day and part of the night as I usually did, I was not preparing proper food for myself. This began to take its toll on my strength, so I began eating at the small restaurant up the street from my office. I went to dinner about nine o'clock one evening, then directly home and to bed. Before the eleven o'clock news came on television I was so ill I drove myself to the hospital emergency room. My stomach ache had thrown my whole body into near crisis condition. The doctors gave me some kind of effervescent solution to drink and as soon as it was down it acted like a new broom, it swept my stomach clean. I received an injection for pain and a friend who worked in the emergency room drove me back home. I went back to bed, slept off the heavy sedation and went to work the next morning. Two weeks later I received a vacation with pay and decided to drive to Kentucky to join my wife and baby for a visit with her parents and some much-needed rest. I was always in need of rest.

I was looking forward to this visit with much anxiety, therefore, drove my car into destruction. About two hundred miles from her home my motor caught fire and was burned beyond repair. An alley mechanic the state trooper sent out to tow me in led me on for half the night letting me think he could repair it and I could be on my way again soon. I was exhausted from having worked all week then starting out on my drive without rest. I stood outside for hours in the dewy night, then sat in the back seat of the car to try to relax. I got no relaxation. My whole body became stiff and I could feel pain down my back and

legs. I knew I must get away from there so I took a bus to
Ashland.

My family was shocked when they saw me walking
down the street from the bus station. It took me some time
to explain that I had not had an accident. We returned to
St. Louis by plane. I made arrangements with some man
that had towed my car off the highway to bring it to St.
Louis. When he arrived the car was just another clump of
junk, enroute it had broken the tow chain and was destroyed by an oncoming truck. The tow driver still wanted
pay for this. At the rate my blood pressure had gone up
when I saw the car he was lucky I did not become violent.
Every fiber of me ached with anger. I do not know how
many pain pills I took to avoid an attack from that anger
and anxiety. The pains pressed me unbearably for hours. I
learned from that incident to hold tighter reins on my emotions. I tried hard to avoid angry confrontations; therefore,
have taken some insults many men would have committed
murder for. This had been difficult for me since I have always had a violent temper. My temper grew into a shield
in later years in order to keep people whom I thought
would upset me at a safe distance.

*I have had a reasonably long vacation from the hospi-
tal at this time but I can feel my time running out. I have
constant pain in my ribs and a blinding headache, not the
kind of headache one takes a Stanback for, but the skull
and facial bones ache.*

After some week wrestling with the discomfort I went
to see my doctor. He calmly said, "Clarence if I didn't know
you and your wife so well I would say you are a stupid
man, I am sure you have pneumonia in one side, maybe
both. I am going to get you a bed at the hospital this very
minute."

I told him I had some very important business to take
care of and that I would go to the hospital the next morn-

ing. He reluctantly agreed. Before the night was over I wished a thousand times I had gone when he had suggested. I kept my wife up all night making cold orange juice, lemonade and anything else we had she could put cracked ice into. My temperature was so high and pain so severe I thought this must surely be the end. My breathing was so difficult I woke the people in the downstairs apartments. I felt as though I would smother any minute. My friend, Paul Chamber, came and practically carried me bodily to his car and took me to the hospital. The doctor in the receiving room sent me quickly to a room and started oxygen. He must have forgotten the pain injection because the deeper I breathed, the more painful my rib cage became; the pains were shooting like arrows from the spinal column and crashing together in the middle of my sternum. I was solely tempted to scream out until the pain was relieved or I passed out; either would have been better than what I had.

Mari was very disturbed she had only seen my have one big one before. It was hard for her to understand how I had lived through many as bad and some worse. I repeat, there is no way to give anyone who has not had sickle-cell anemia any idea of the devastating pain nor the stifling after-effects. She understood better when a doctor told her the pain was more severe than giving birth without sedation.

My wife was subjected to many anxious moments in those early years of our marriage, with a young child and my frequent illness, there was always something to keep her at disadvantage. I suffered in silence many times in order to avoid undue concern for her. I still do.

Three years have gone by now, I have moved my family to Detroit, Michigan. The weather here is very different from that of St. Louis. The long cold winters, the ever-present snow and winter rains are a menace to me. There are many days I don't get comfortable until I take my nightly hot bath, even though I wear the heaviest thermal drawers I can find. I did not realize the weather was so hard here; I negotiated a change because the hours I am compelled to work are about half of what I had there and the salary is double. I also am able to do a bit of moonlighting if necessary. I could not do that in St. Louis; there weren't enough hours in the day to take care of the one position. I required undivided attention.

After a few months in Detroit I began to shed some of the tension from my mind and body. I was not exposed to sixteen-and eighteen-hour shifts; I had only one eight-hour shift embalming. I still had leg ulcers but was not on my feet as long as before. I was able to discontinue the strong pain medication to a great degree. Many days I only took Anacin or aspirin. This did not alter the fact I still had some pain daily but brought it to a tolerance level. For about fourteen months after coming from St. Louis to Detroit, things went considerably well with me. I was fortunate in not having to be hospitalized. I really did not have a regular doctor for a while. I did for myself. Most of the medications needed to dress a leg ulcer could be bought at the corner drugstore.

Mari became ill and was hospitalized twice in 1965 and my having to take care of the baby and carry out my duties on my job put some extra pressure on me, physically and mentally. By the time I finished work, picked Kimberly up from my sister-in-law's home, gave her dinner and a bath, I was thoroughly exhausted. During this time my leg ulcer was reactivated. Then I struck it with the hearse door. It became unbearable so quickly that my wife had to sign out of the hospital so that I could go in the next day. My brother James came over to take me. I was very ill when I reached the hospital, but the doctors there did not know what I was talking about when I told them I had sickle-cell anemia. One said to me, "You do not have to pretend to be that sick to get in, you do have a temperature, so we will admit you and check you out tomorrow."

98

When I asked for an injection for pain the doctor asked
how long I had been taking hard drugs. I tried hard not to
let myself become upset, but was prodded so long and un-
necessarily with lame-brained questions until I lost control.
When he sat down on a stool in front of me, my stomach
did an upside down and I threw up everything I had eaten
for the last three days up all over him. He then gave me
morphine and sent me to bed. That shot did not last very
long. Four hours later I was about ready to climb every
wall I could see. I asked to take a hot bath but was refused
because no orders were left that would permit it. I was de-
nied about everything I asked for during that first long
night but I survived it in spite of that.

The next day I was transferred to another room. No
one got any sleep that night because the orderly was changing my linen so often. I perspired freely because of the
morphine.

I think I was poked and questioned by at least twenty-
five young doctors during the next three or four days. I
soon found I knew more about sickle-cell anemia than they
did. I was a novelty to them. According to what they knew
of the disease I was not even supposed to be there. I was
supposed to be in the cemetery. I told them I was sorry if
my presence there exploded their theories. They took so
many blood samples that I had to have a transfusion. I became so ill in the days that followed that everyone thought
this would be the last one I would live to tell about. The
first thing Mari would do was listen to see if I was still
grunting and groaning, before she came in. She would be
afraid, if she did not hear me, that I was gone for sure. My
pains became so hard until the doctors had to give me
morphine intravenously. I became frightened because this
is a very dangerous process. I could feel my heart flutter
and skip like a radio with static or a shortage in the wiring.
I was very ill for weeks. I had never been directly confined
to bed for eight weeks as I was this time. Many of those
early days I did not know the difference between the day or

night exept somewhere along the way they put out the lights. I was too weary to eat. I lost eighteen pounds.

My little family was having a rough time getting around because of the awful winter weather that year. They were not used to all the snow and zero weather. I began worrying about them and the doctor gave me tranquilizers so that I did not become too upset. I was barely able to come home before Christmas. Due to my low blood count my leg was still sore. Previously when I was in the hospital it generally healed all by itself, but not so this time. I left the hospital depending heavily on a cane. I found it necessary to return to work immediately. There was no income unless I did.

Stinson Funeral Home bought a stool tall enough for me to sit on, even at the preparation table, and I learned to do as much work that way as anyone could do with two good legs. I was given a good year-end bonus by the Stinson Funeral Home for meritorious service that year.

During the years that followed my attacks became lighter and further apart—some severe discomfort but not hospitalizing. I have been right on the brink of immobilization many times with leg ulcers but hung on through prayer and sheer willpower. I have done nearly six hundred cases a year for several years since my last hospitalization. Some of those years I did not miss a single day at work because of sickle-cell anemia.

I will not lead you to believe I have beaten the monster. I will not say I have walked out of the darkness of pain into the light of freedom from suffering.

There are many days and nights of the same old horror, but after all the bouts I have fought, I have learned the battle plans of SCA: I try to slug it before it slugs me. I do not believe those few who are familiar with my battles would want a refund.

I, too, believe I have fought well. Ten years have passed since I was hospitalized. My health seems to improve with age.